Microbiology for Clinicians

Microbiology for Clinicians

R. N. Grüneberg, MD, FRCPath.
Consultant Microbiologist
University College Hospital
London WC1E 6AU

University Park Press
Baltimore

Published in USA and Canada by
University Park Press
300 North Charles Street
Baltimore, Maryland 21201

Published in UK by
MTP Press Limited
Falcon House
Lancaster, England

ISBN 0-8391-1682-9

LCC 81-50285

Printed in Great Britain

This book is dedicated to Dr E. Joan Stokes

Contents

	Foreword	9
1	Microbes and man	11
2	The bacteriology laboratory	21
3	Viruses, fungi and parasites	41
4	Antibacterial drugs	59
5	Infections in general practice	85
6	Infections in hospitals	99
7	Control of infection in the community	115
8	Control of infection in hospitals	133
9	The control of antibiotic resistance	151
10	Medical microbiology in the future	165
	References	173
	Index	175

Foreword

A practising clinician is required to use knowledge from many different fields. It is unrealistic to expect him to be master of more than a few. In reality, clinicians acquire a smattering of information on most relevant subjects, and learn which texts provide the detailed information which is occasionally required on more highly specialized matters. In my professional contacts with clinicians and medical students it has become evident that they often lack the simple framework of microbiological knowledge necessary to guide their actions. This is because standard textbooks and learned treatises alike are concerned with imparting a body of information rather than with presenting what the doctor needs to know in order to manage his patients.

This volume is an attempt to help clinicians in their everyday practice. To that end I have kept it short and have not dwelt at length even on those topics which especially interest me. No attempt has been made to write a textbook: many of these already exist. A few references are given to major reviews and to sources justifying some of the more forthright statements. The subject of medical microbiology is broad and involved. I have therefore seen it as my task to simplify the presentation of the material, being very selective with regard to content and giving my own views on matters of clinical significance. I hope that, despite occasional divergences of opinion from those presented here, the reader will find this book easy to read and helpful in clinical practice.

Although I accept responsibility for the opinions expressed in this book, I am grateful to my colleagues for their support and for giving me their valuable time. Constructive criticism, initially resented, but subsequently accepted with gratitude, came from Mr A. W. F. Cremer, Dr R. J. Hay, Dr Anne Grüneberg, Mr B. J. Mellars, Dr G. L. Ridgway, Dr D. S. Ridley, Dr E. J. Stokes and Dr Mair E. M. Thomas. I am indebted to Mr P. Luton for the photographs, and to Mrs A. A. Luton for splendid secretarial support.

1

Microbes and man

There shall no evil happen unto thee: neither shall any plague come nigh thy
  dwelling.
For he shall give his angels charge over thee: to keep thee in all thy ways.
Psalms xci, 2

Microbes are not popular. This is perhaps not surprising, considering
the historical background from which our knowledge of microbes
arises. Nonetheless, this view of micro-organisms as mediators of
death and disaster is largely inappropriate.

Even those bacteria which are capable of causing disease in man may
only do so semi-accidentally. Very few organisms are obligate human
parasites: the large majority are commensals, normally causing no
trouble, and capable of becoming pathogenic only under unusual
circumstances.

Historical perspective

Tens of thousands of years ago, man lived in wandering groups of
quite small size. Under such circumstances, it is probable that he
suffered no more microbial disease than would, say, a pack of wolves
now. Individuals would contract infections from time to time and
would either recover or die. The possibilities of spread of infection to
other individuals were limited. Since the group was on the move, the
opportunities for accumulation of pathogenic microbes through pollu-

11

tion of water or food supply were minimal, and there was probably little contact between human tribes before the beginning of settled habitation.

Later, when man began to settle and to farm rather than to hunt, new problems were posed in what we now call public health. Man began to eat new foods, to tend flocks which might themselves become infected, and to become dependent on them for his food supply. Gradually, his settled communities became larger and provided new opportunities for spread of infection. The arrangements for disposing of waste and for maintaining a pure water supply became more and more inadequate as communities increased in size. As they grew from hamlets to villages, to small towns and then to cities, these problems grew worse and overcrowding, filth and malnutrition became endemic.

We know from our own experience in modern cities that when a city population is well fed and well housed in clean, spacious circumstances, and when care is taken about purity of water and food supplies, and about the disposal of sewage and other waste, serious human infection is a rarity. Nonetheless, this happy state of affairs is relatively new. Until only a century or two ago, urban populations were subject to endemic tuberculosis, smallpox, diphtheria, cholera, typhoid and typhus. From time to time, great epidemics of plague would decimate or destroy large populations. When it became clear in the mid-nineteenth century that these contagions were caused by microbes, the population took an unfriendly view of their tiny neighbours which now seems to be unjustified. The problems were not really caused by the microbes, but by man. Microbial diseases were merely a symptom of the degradation of man resulting from disorganized urbanization: they were not its cause. It could be argued that if it had not been for the infectious diseases, man might still be living in mediaeval urban squalor.

Major outbreaks of infectious diseases resulting in a high death rate are very unusual, although they continue to colour our collective view of the nature of contagion. To be successful, a human pathogen should adopt a strategy of causing minimum lasting damage to its host while providing a living for itself and facilitating its spread from man to man. A pathogen which destroys all its hosts will have great difficulty in spreading from one to the next. At the same time, a human population exposed to a new microbial threat of great potency will gradually select from its survivors a population with greater resistance to the threat. These two interacting factors of decreasing virulence of the parasite and increasing hardiness of the host, bring about changes in the nature of infection.

Such changes may be very rapid or more gradual. An example of rapid change is that which has occurred in human infection caused by the Group A haemolytic streptococci in the course of the last human generation. Scarlet fever, for instance, used to be a much-feared, often fatal infection. Nowadays, haemolytic streptococcal infection is rarer and usually more mild. This effect is not a reflection of the use of penicillin. There is no certainty that rapid changes such as this will be maintained. An example of more gradual change is that of pneumonic or bubonic plague. The great outbreaks of plague in the cities of Europe in the fourteenth and seventeenth centuries struck with such savagery as to kill perhaps a third of the population of the continent on each occasion. The modern form of these diseases causes isolated rural cases of infection, usually with a more insidious course.

The value of long exposure of human populations to their familiar infections is most readily seen when they meet new, unfamiliar pathogens. Examples are numerous, and include the high death rates of Australian aborigines and Pacific islanders from imported measles and tuberculosis; the impact of imported New World syphilis on the population of Europe, and the effect of malaria and other fevers on Europeans visiting West Africa (the 'white man's grave').

Nowadays, infections are usually sporadic and mild, and only rarely do they spread over wide areas. The most striking example of such spread in recent times, is the epidemic and even pandemic spread of influenza to which there may be little human herd resistance because of antigenic variation on the part of the influenza virus. There were said to be more deaths due to the great influenza pandemic after the first world war than to the four years of the war itself, despite its reputation as the most bloody in human history. The association here between pestilence, war and famine is a recurrent theme. Whenever communities are disrupted by the damage inflicted by war and consequent starvation, epidemics become more likely. Similarly, a single human being becomes a more ready prey to intercurrent infection when debilitated (e.g. by malnutrition, injury, or recent infection).

Folk memories of the horrors of the mass epidemics of previous centuries die very hard. An echo of this comes to us from the prominence given in the newspapers, on radio and on television to the details of the occasional cases of typhoid fever diagnosed in Western Europe, usually in travellers returning from abroad. It is implied by this that such cases, if not vigorously contained, represent a serious threat to the public health. This is just not true. More exotic imports such as Lassa fever create near panic, probably inappropriately.

The triumphs of the early microbiologists such as Pasteur, Lister, and Koch in recognizing the microbial nature of infectious diseases, led to the virtual elimination of many of the more serious human epidemic or endemic infections. They also gave rise to a public misapprehension that the activities of microbes are wholly baleful and that the only good germ is a dead germ. This is manifest nonsense.

A balanced relationship

The vast majority of micro-organisms have nothing to do with disease in man. They live in the soil, in vegetable matter, in water, in plants and in animals. They fix nitrogen; degrade dead biological material; ferment fruit, producing alcohol and vinegar; give taste to foodstuffs, and so on. Only infrequently do the many organisms capable of causing infection in man actually do so. The bowel commensal *Escherichia coli* occasionally causes human urinary tract infection. Nonetheless, a single gram of human faeces may contain 10^6-10^8 individuals. The human bowel may contain a kilogram of faeces with a population of 10^9-10^{11} *E. coli* organisms and the bowel flora of all 4 000 000 000 living human beings may contain $10^{18}-10^{20}$. Multiplying by ten to allow for those in non-human sites gives an approximate total of 10^{20} *E. coli* individuals in existence at any one time. Under ideal circumstances, these organisms have a generation time of approximately 20 minutes. A single human generation (say 30 years) therefore contains about 750 000 generations of *E. coli*. About 15% of all human beings probably develop a urinary tract infection with *E. coli* at some time in their lives. The chances against any one individual *E. coli* causing this are therefore approximately 10^{16} to 1. Such figures suggest that it is scarcely reasonable to regard *E. coli* as a pathogen at all. Clearly its propensity for causing harm to man is very slight, and it only becomes a pathogen under most unusual circumstances.

It is also true that man's normal microbial flora protects him from invasion by other microbes. This is seen most clearly when the use of broad spectrum antibiotics clears the usual antibiotic-sensitive commensal flora away and permits overgrowth of resistant organisms which are usually present only in small numbers, enabling these to invade the tissues. Examples include staphylococcal enterocolitis in patients given tetracyclines following gastric surgery, candidal vaginitis following the use of ampicillin, and antibiotic associated colitis. The mechanisms through which this protection is mediated are not entirely clear. Probably, it is achieved for the most part by producing a local micro-environment disagreeable to other organisms, through altering the pH, the concentration of some metabolite, or the oxygen tension. Some organisms also elaborate diffusible chemicals, bacteriocines, capable of preventing locally the growth of other strains of the same species.

The untold multitudes of microbes covering each and every one of us internally and externally coexist with each other and with us in a very complicated and constantly changing way. They are dependent upon each other and upon us, and we are dependent upon them. Were it possible for us to destroy all our microbial fellow travellers (and it is not) we would damage our own interests very profoundly. The problems of doing any such thing are compounded by two major factors. The first concerns the very different natures and needs of the many kinds of microbes, and the second the vast capacity of microorganisms to change their genetic properties in the face of metabolic challenge such as the development of a new antibiotic. Bacteria, for example, are not only vastly more numerous than man (by a factor of perhaps 10^{20}) but they produce their generations much more quickly. The prophet Abraham lived about 120 human generations ago, during which time there has been opportunity for perceptible genetic change to occur in man (at least as seen by man himself). The equivalent bacterial genetic time scale is about 40 hours, and much larger populations are involved. Additionally, the metabolic processes of bacteria and of man are not so very different and nor are the materials from which they are composed. Any attempt at complete eradication of the bacteria would therefore probably also lead to the eradication of their human host.

In any case, our only legitimate interests in this direction lie in attempting to prevent human infection and, when this fails, in attempting to eradicate only the microbial invaders, not the whole microbial flora. Many of the worst therapeutic disasters follow from attempts to do more than this.

Microbes and disease

As has already been indicated, there are relatively few microbes so specialized that they can live only at our expense. An example of such specialization is the bacterium *Neisseria gonorrhoeae* (the causative agent of gonorrhoea) which is pathogenic only to man. A viral example is the smallpox virus. The fact that smallpox has no host other than man was the key to its eradication. When such organisms are recognized in specimens from patients in the laboratory there is no intellectual problem in attributing a pathogenic rôle to them.

There are other organisms which, while pathogenic only to man, are also capable of survival outside the human body. An example of this is *Salmonella typhi*, the causative agent of typhoid fever, which, while causing a distinctive human disease, may also be isolated from sewage, foodstuffs and water supplies. It is possible to isolate this organism in the laboratory from specimens both from patients with typhoid fever and from those who had the disease long ago. These latter, asymptomatic, carriers of *S. typhi* are not ill, but represent a possible source of infection to others. It is logically quite possible for such a carrier to be suffering from another illness. This creates an obvious difficulty in the interpretation of laboratory findings.

There are also microbes which have a pathogenic rôle both in man and in other animals. *Brucella abortus* and *Brucella melitensis* cause brucellosis in man, and also cause 'spontaneous abortion' in cattle and goats, respectively. The presence of these organisms in human material is indicative of disease. However, some infectious organisms are shared between man and animals and can be isolated from either, both when in a state of good health and when diseased. Examples are to be found among the intestinal pathogens of the genus *Salmonella*. Again, the mere laboratory isolation of a potential pathogen from human material does not necessarily imply the presence, at that time, of disease caused by that organism.

Much more common nowadays than any of the situations so far described, is the identification of non-specific infections capable of being caused by any of a range of potential pathogens most of which are commonly or usually commensals in man. Medical microbiology in industrialized societies has moved away from the specific, named fevers with a single pathogen (such as diphtheria, caused by *Coryne-bacterium diphtheriae* or plague caused by *Yersinia (Pasteurella) pestis*), or with only two or three pathogens (such as enteric fever caused by *S. typhi* or *S. paratyphi*, or cholera caused by *Vibrio cholerae* or its el Tor biotype). These societies are now more concerned with respiratory infections, meningitis, and urinary tract infections each of which may be caused by many different types of organism, giving rise to very similar clinical features. In less prosperous societies, although these latter conditions also occur, the named fevers such as yellow fever, diphtheria, plague and cholera still play a large part in human disease.

In the nineteenth century, the principles under which it was possible to assign a pathogenic rôle to an organism were clearly stated, and are known to us in modified form as Koch's Postulates:

(1)   It must be possible to grow the organism in the laboratory.
(2)   The organism must be isolated from all cases of the disease.
(3)   It must not be isolated from those who do not have the disease.
(4)   It must be capable of causing the disease in a susceptible animal.

The principles were invaluable at the time of their introduction in finding out which organisms caused which diseases. However, there were problems.

(1)   The leprosy bacillus *Mycobacterium leprae* and the organism of syphilis *Treponema pallidum* cannot be grown in the laboratory.
(2)   The pathogen cannot be isolated from all cases of human brucellosis (the diagnosis often depending on the identification of an antibody response to the pathogen).
(3)   As it has already been indicated, asymptomatic carriage of

Salmonella typhi (which under other circumstances causes typhoid fever) may occur.

(4)   Some human pathogens (e.g. smallpox virus), have no known susceptible animal hosts*.

Even with the specific infectious diseases, therefore, the requirements of Koch's Postulates often cannot be fulfilled completely and they can much more rarely be complied with in the non-specific infections which cause the majority of infectious conditions in developed countries.

Nowadays, it is more clearly seen that the microbial world cannot be arbitrarily divided into those organisms which are, and those organisms which are not, pathogenic to man. What we now recognize is that there is a spectrum of organisms from those which are very pathogenic, through those which are occasional pathogens, to those which very rarely cause human disease. There is almost no organism which cannot, on occasion, cause human illness. Moreover, the full range of infectious diseases in man has by no means been explored. Quite apart from the periodic recognition of 'new' tropical fevers (some with very disagreeable features such as Lassa fever, Marburg disease or Ebola fever), new infectious diseases of temperate climates continue to be revealed. Recent examples include the appearance of enteritis caused by rotaviruses; the realization that the commonest cause of infectious diarrhoea is *Campylobacter* enteritis; the emergence of *Clostridium difficile* as a cause of antibiotic associated colitis, and the sensational appearance of a new form of pneumonia, Legionnaire's disease, caused by a newly recognized organism, *Legionella pneumophila*. Moreover, the nature of the infectious diseases has changed, is changing, and will continue to change.

Before going on, in the next chapter, to consider laboratory methods, and how the laboratory should be used to investigate communicable diseases, there remains to be discussed the major problem of the distinction between infection and colonization.

---

* The diligence of the search for susceptible hosts for research purposes has been remarkable: note the use of the armadillo as a susceptible host for the leprosy bacillus, *Mycobacterium leprae*, the chimpanzee for hepatitis viruses, and the use of inoculation of material from Buruli ulcer containing *Mycobacterium ulcerans* into the foot pad of the mouse.

Infection and colonization

We now know that almost any micro-organism may cause human disease, but how do we know whether a particular isolate is causing infection or if it is merely co-existing with its host? Failure to draw this distinction results in much avoidable friction between clinicians and laboratory workers, and a great deal of unnecessary, and possibly harmful, treatment of patients.

Organisms may cause infection by giving rise to local sepsis (inflammation), by causing a spreading infection in continuity, by giving rise to blood borne infection, by causing immunological damage locally or at a distance, or by elaborating toxins which may themselves be harmful to man. These effects are all detectable clinically in varying degree. Every medical student is taught that infection is a major cause of inflammation, and that the signs of inflammation are redness, swelling, pain, fever and loss of function. In general, therefore, infection is a *clinical diagnosis*. When it is suspected, a prudent clinician will despatch appropriate specimens for bacteriological examination. A competent laboratory will then report what it finds to be present, and this, under ideal circumstances, will correspond with the microbial flora of the site sampled. The assessment of which of the organisms isolated by the laboratory may be relevant to the patient's condition is a *clinical decision*.

The laboratory can provide some clues to aid this clinical assessment. If direct microscopy of the clinical material shows the presence of pus cells, this is evidence of an inflammatory response. If a mixed growth shows a predominance of one type, this suggests that greater weight should be given to that organism, particularly if it is also present predominantly in the direct microscopic examination. If the microbe reported is a well known pathogen in the appropriate site, this should also be given due (but no more) weight.

In the absence of clinical signs of infection, microbiology laboratory reports, no matter how terrifying they sound, should be treated with reserve. The basic principle is that the doctor should treat the patient and not the laboratory report. It also follows that, under most circumstances, it is wise not to take specimens for microbiological examination unless there is evidence of infection. Organisms isolated from sites without evidence of infection should be regarded as commensals which are merely colonizing the sites, and should be ignored. This is not to suggest that the 'carrier state' of some organisms such as *Salmonella typhi* or *Neisseria meningitidis* is of no consequence, only that the implications of its presence are different from those of the recognition of the disease state caused by the same organisms.

2

The bacteriology laboratory

> The Microbe is so very small
> You cannot make him out at all,
> But many sanguine people hope
> To see him through a microscope.
> His jointed tongue that lies beneath
> A hundred curious rows of teeth;
> His seven tufted tails with lots
> Of lovely pink and purple spots,
> On each of which a pattern stands,
> Composed of forty separate bands;
> His eyebrows of a tender green;
> All these have never yet been seen —
> But Scientists, who ought to know,
> Assure us that they must be so . . .
> Oh! let us never, never doubt
> What nobody is sure about!

The Microbe, Hilaire Belloc (1870—1953)

In this chapter I propose to give a brief summary of the distinctive features of the bacteria and their classification; an outline of the nature of relevant laboratory classification techniques; some comments on specimen collection and handling, and an outline of how infectious conditions should be investigated. Those requiring a detailed exposition of any of these topics are referred to the standard works.

21

A similar treatment of the special features of viruses, fungi and parasites is given in Chapter 3.

The bacteria

These are unicellular organisms ranging in size from 0.5 to 5 μm, and are usually capable of independent growth. They contain both DNA and RNA and usually replicate by binary fission. Some strains can produce hardy resting phases called spores, capable of resuming multiplication after lengthy dormant periods. Many bacteria are motile, often by virtue of the possession of whip-like structures called flagella. Most species have rigid cell walls. Overlying the cell wall there may be a capsule. The genetic material is concentrated in a single ring-shaped chromosome. Sometimes, separate small pieces of DNA are detectable. Granules of various kinds may be present in the cytoplasm.

The rigid cell wall of a bacterium gives it one of several shapes: it may be rod-shaped (bacillus), rounded (coccus), comma-shaped (vibrio) or corkscrew-shaped (spirochaete). The cell walls may or may not retain various dyes under standard conditions, so providing a basis for differentiation (Gram-positive or Gram-negative). Some bacterial cell walls have chemical characteristics such that they will retain dyes even when attempts are made to leach them out with acid or alcohol.

The growth requirements of bacteria are varied. With the exception of a very few (e.g. *Chlamydia* spp.), they do not require living cells for replication, and can therefore be grown in the laboratory on simple organic media. *Chlamydia* spp. can be grown in tissue cultures. Most medically important bacteria are not particularly demanding in their growth requirements but a few, such as those without rigid cell walls (e.g. *Mycoplasma* spp., ureaplasmas and protoplasts), do require special conditions. Bacteria will survive and grow in very varied temperatures, some being attuned to survival in polar waters and others to the conditions in naturally occurring hot springs at just under 100 °C. Most of the medically important bacteria have growth optima at around the human body temperature (37 °C), but there is some variation around this temperature. For example, *Campylobacter jejuni* grows well *in vitro* at 42 °C while *Mycobacterium ulcerans* does better at 28–31 °C.

The optimum atmospheric conditions for bacterial growth show wide variation from those of obligate aerobes at one end of the spectrum to those of obligate anaerobes at the other. The many intermediates, such as facultative anaerobes and micro-aerophilic bacteria, require something in between. Many bacteria grow better with added carbon dioxide in a humid atmosphere. Most bacteria are quite tolerant of changes in the acidity or alkalinity of their environment, but the medically important strains thrive at or around the pH of human tissues.

The bacteria derive their nutritional needs from organic materials in their environment and have elaborated many enzymes in order to be able to split carbohydrates and other substrates. An analysis of bacterial enzyme production is used in microbial identification. The release of volatile fatty acids as a result of microbial activity may also be used as a diagnostic tool (e.g. gas—liquid chromatography for anaerobes in pus). Some bacteria require special growth factors (X and V factors for *Haemophilus* spp., for example) and there is widely varying susceptibility to growth inhibitors such as bile salts. These variations form part of the identification techniques used in the laboratory.

Some bacteria produce pigments of various colours. The staphylococci were originally classified by their production of gold, lemon yellow or white pigmented colonies. *Serratia marcescens* sometimes produces blood red colonies. Many strains of *Pseudomonas aeruginosa* produce very intense green, fluorescent pyocyanin which diffuses into the medium and may produce green colouration of pus or sputum.

Some bacteria produce various poisonous substances. These are either contained within the organism (endotoxins) or are diffusible (exotoxins). These toxins may produce disease in man or animals independently of the presence of living bacteria.

Various components of bacteria or bacterial products may give rise to an immune response in man or in other animals, causing the production of specific or semi-specific antibodies against a whole range of bacterial antigens. These bacterial antigens are present in cell walls (somatic, or O antigens), in capsules (capsular, or K antigens), in the flagella of motile strains (flagellar, or H antigens), in the whiskery fimbriae which project from the cell walls of many species (fimbrial antigens) and in toxins. This antigenic property of bacteria and bacterial products has some prophylactic and therapeutic importance (see Chapter 7) and provides a laboratory tool for the identification and differentiation of bacteria. Purified preparations of bacterial antigens can be used to test for production, in the patient, of antibodies to similar antigens from invading pathogens, thus providing useful diagnostic information. Antibodies raised against bacterial antigens may immobilize the bacteria but seldom neutralize or inactivate them. Thus, many of the antibodies produced against infecting bacteria are not in any way protective.

Most bacteria, particularly the Gram-negative bacilli, die quickly if removed from a moist environment. However, spore-producing bacteria may survive under dry conditions for months or years, and many Gram-positive organisms will survive without moisture for weeks. Not all bacteria are killed readily by disinfectants and some even grow well in the presence of the weaker formulations. This has implications in the field of infection prevention, and may also be used in the laboratory as a selective means of recovering certain organisms. *Pseudomonas aeruginosa*, for example, will grow well on media containing cetrimide.

Bacteria multiply at varying speeds: coliform organisms have a generation time of 20 minutes or so, while *Mycobacterium tuberculosis* doubles its numbers in about 8 hours. Most of the medically important bacteria have generation times of 20–30 minutes *in vitro* and rather longer *in vivo*. The limiting factors to bacterial growth *in vitro* are exhaustion of food supplies and accumulation of toxic metabolic waste products, the latter often accompanied by inhibitory shifts of pH.

The mode of replication is usually asexual (binary fission) each bacterium dividing into two daughter cells with the same genetic potential as the parent cell. Much more rarely, bacteria 'mate' (conjugate) and the genetic material of the donor cell is transferred into the recipient cell which then divides into two daughter cells each reflecting the genetic constitution of both parents. Conjugation may take place between members of different species or genera, thus implying an enormous capacity for rapid genetic change among the bacteria. The process of bacterial spore production manifested by some species, is not a reproductive mechanism but a strategy for survival under unpromising conditions.

The genetic material of bacteria is largely concentrated in the single ring-shaped chromosome. A small number of additional, non-chromosomally integrated pieces of DNA (plasmids) may also be present in the cytoplasm. In binary fission, the ring chromosome is replicated and the daughter cells each receive one of the duplicated chromosomes plus a share of any plasmids present. At conjugation the recipient cell receives the donor's DNA, whether chromosomal or not, and, at subsequent binary fission, the daughter cells receive some from each parent. Two other mechanisms of bacterium to bacterium transfer of genetic material may occur. These are called transduction and transformation. In transduction pieces of chromosomal or extra-chromosomal (plasmid) DNA are carried accidentally from one host bacterium to another by the migration of a bacterial virus. These bacterial viruses are called bacteriophages and react with their bacterial hosts either by replicating within them and then bursting them in order to pass to the next host cell (lytic bacteriophages), or by integrating their viral genetic material with the bacterial chromosome and passing with the bacterial DNA to successive generations of bacterial cells (temperate, or lysogenic bacteriophages). The effects of this latter phenomenon of lysogeny are varied since the presence of the 'phage DNA may alter the characteristics of the host bacterium. This is the case with *Corynebacterium diphtheriae* which produces only local effects (sore throat, oedema of the fauces) in man unless it is lysogenized by a particular strain of bacteriophage. When this occurs, the bacterium produces a very potent exotoxin which results in the development of the systemic effects of diphtheria. The accidental carriage of bacterial DNA from one cell to another by 'phage mediated transduction may transfer various properties including resistance to antibiotics. This mechanism is most important with Gram-positive organisms such as the staphylococci.

In transformation, dividing bacteria assimilate pieces of free bacterial DNA present in the environment and incorporate them into their own chromosome with the consequent possibility of significant genetic change. This phenomenon affects the pneumococci, but is otherwise rare in nature although it can be induced experimentally.

Transfer of genetic material in bacteria by binary fission, conjugation and transduction (but not by transformation) added to the effects on these, as on all other living organisms, of mutation contributes to the rich variability and rapid adaptability of bacteria.

Classification of bacteria

The bacteria are classified, as are other organisms, using the Linnaean binomial system. The details of the methods used and of the constantly changing nomenclature are not important in the present context, but interested readers will gain some insight into the problems by reference to a standard laboratory manual of bacterial identification such as that by Cowan and Steel (1974). For our present purpose, it is possible to use a very much simplified classification of the bacterial genera using only three characteristics: shape of the organism, staining reactions, and whether the organism is aerobic or anaerobic. By these means it is possible to divide the medically important bacterial genera into groups as shown in Table 1. Within these groups the identification of parti-

Table 1   Simple classification of medically important bacterial genera

Bacterial shape	Staining properties	Aerobic or anaerobic	Genera
Bacilli (rods)	Gram-positive	aerobic	*Bacillus, Corynebacterium, Listeria*
		anaerobic	*Actinomyces, Clostridium, Lactobacillus* (microaerophilic)
	Gram-negative	aerobic	*Bordetella, Brucella, Citrobacter, Enterobacter, Escherichia, Haemophilus, Klebsiella, Pasteurella, Proteus, Providencia, Pseudomonas, Salmonella, Shigella, Yersinia* (*Pasteurella*)
		anaerobic	*Bacteroides, Fusiformis*
	Acid fast	aerobic	*Mycobacterium*
Vibrios (commas)	Gram-negative	aerobic	*Campylobacter, Vibrio*
Cocci	Gram-positive	aerobic	*Micrococcus, Staphylococcus, Streptococcus*
		anaerobic	*Peptococcus, Peptostreptococcus*
	Gram-negative	aerobic	*Neisseria*
		anaerobic	*Veillonella*
Spirochaetes			*Leptospira, Treponema*

cular genera and species involves detailed cultural, biochemical and serological testing.

As Table 1 shows, it is possible to begin to classify bacteria grown in the laboratory with only minimal information about the microscopic appearance of the organisms, their Gram-staining characteristics, and whether they grow in air or anaerobically. The detailed laboratory classification should then follow a systematic process of sequential analytical steps culminating in final identification. Usually identification as far as the species suffices, but sometimes the process must go further in order to discriminate between different strains of a species.

In practice, the systematic process is rarely adhered to in detail. This is partly because very precise identification of bacteria is not often clinically necessary, and partly because an experienced microbiologist can use his skill to cut out unnecessary steps. A professional zoologist may know how to establish beyond doubt that a particular creature is an elephant but rarely troubles to do so because he knows one when he sees it. Similarly, an experienced microbiologist may look at the colonies growing on various commonly used culture media and have little doubt about the identity of many of the more usual bacteria, at least as far as their genera. A very few confirmatory tests will then enable him to complete the identification as far as species or even beyond.

After the initial morphological and cultural tests, the next process is to study the chemical activities of the test organism. Does it ferment various carbohydrates (with or without the production of gas)? Does it grow in the presence of bile salts? Is it susceptible to this chemical, or that? Does it liquefy gelatin, or does it split hydrogen peroxide? The application of such standard chemical tests may be sufficient to complete the identification. If not, the next stage will be an antigenic analysis using specific antisera, raised in animals, against particular bacterial antigens. This may be relatively simple as in the identification of haemolytic streptococci by Lancefield's grouping, or may be exceedingly complicated. The guidebook (the Kauffmann—White scheme) to the serological analysis of the many hundred different serotypes (species) in the genus *Salmonella*, for example, is a substantial volume.

Sometimes it is necessary, usually for epidemiological reasons, to identify individual strains of an organism within a species. This may be done in several different ways: for example, by antigenic analysis, by bacteriophage typing or by bacteriocine production. Different methods have been elaborated for various organisms. For *Escherichia coli*, for example, serotyping is used. Some 160 different somatic (O) antigens, 90 capsular (K) antigens and 49 flagellar (H) antigens have been described. By testing extracts of the unknown *E. coli* strain against specific O, K and H antisera, the organism can be assigned to a particular O:K:H serotype distinguishing it from other serotypes of that species. Strains of *Staphylococcus aureus* (pyogenes) may be differentiated by their varying susceptibility to lysis by a battery of standard bacteriophages, since susceptibility to lysis by bacterial viruses is strain specific. Other organisms (e.g. *Pseudomonas aeruginosa*) may be classified by their ability to produce diffusible substances (bacteriocines) which inhibit the growth of other strains of the same species. By observing the pattern of inhibition of growth of a standard set of strains of the species concerned caused by the presence of bacteriocines produced by the test organism, it is possible to assign it to a particular bacteriocine group.

These methods of 'fingerprinting' strains of bacteria may be important in clinical research, or in epidemiological studies of the spread of infection, but very rarely affect the management of individual patients.

The work of a clinical bacteriology laboratory

Clinical bacteriology laboratories have become technological factories handling vast numbers of specimens daily. Since delay decreases the clinical relevance of a report, they are geared to produce approximately correct information rapidly rather than precise answers at leisure. Most of the work done can be divided into two categories: (1) cultural tests and (2) serological tests.

Bacteriological culture work

Specimens for culture are of two fundamental kinds: those from sites which are normally sterile, and those from sites with a normal flora. The methods used for sites which are normally sterile are relatively straightforward, since any organism isolated, even if only in small numbers, may be assumed to be significant unless there is evidence of contamination.

Direct microscopy may be undertaken to see what evidence of inflammation (pus cells, red cells, etc.) is present, and whether any organisms are observable. The results of this direct microscopy may be a useful guide to immediate treatment, as in the case of findings in cerebrospinal fluid from patients with meningitis. Cultures will be set up using a number of clinically relevant organisms, and in a variety of different atmospheres (air, air plus carbon dioxide, anaerobic mixtures). Direct tests of antibiotic sensitivity may also be set up for some types of specimen. After suitable periods of incubation, the cultures are examined for bacterial growth. Isolated bacteria are identified and tested for sensitivity to a range of antibiotics relevant to the clinical circumstances. As soon as findings warrant it, a preliminary report is sent out describing the state of the investigations. The real difficulties with this sort of work lie in recognizing whether a cultured organism is a genuine pathogen or merely a contaminant.

The culture of pathogens from sites with a normal flora is much more difficult: firstly because there may be very few pathogens among a multitude of commensals, and secondly because a satisfactory report depends much more on the judgement of the bench worker than is the case with specimens from normally sterile sites. Different methods are used for different types of specimen. Again, a variety of media and atmospheres is used to cover the range of possible pathogens. Inhibitory substances, including antibiotics, may be used to discourage the growth of commensal organisms and so make it easier to recognize any pathogens. A chemical, such as lactose, may be incorporated into the media and an indicator used to differentiate between colonies able to ferment the chemical and those unable to do so. Bacteria unable to ferment lactose, for example, include intestinal pathogens of the genera *Salmonella* and *Shigella*. From the many types of organism cultured, those which may be pathogenic are selected out. These must then be purified, identified and tested for sensitivity to appropriate antibiotics. This selection of the potentially relevant organisms requires great skill and judgement on the part of the culture plate reader. Reporting everything is just as unhelpful to the clinician as failing to identify the pathogen. Again, the whole process must be completed as quickly as possible if useful information is to be given.

Clinicians often say that they are more interested in the antibiotic sensitivity test results than in the identification of organisms grown in the laboratory. There is some sense in this, but not much. The clinician should be able to assess whether the organism isolated by the laboratory is relevant to his patient's condition, and whether it suggests the need for other measures (e.g. the use of antitoxin in tetanus, or the need for isolation in typhoid, or for contact tracing in gonorrhoea). He should be able to recognize a change in pathogenic bacterial flora in his patient with the passage of time, perhaps reflecting in part the treatment given. More information about antibiotic sensitivity testing and the interpretation of the results is given in Chapter 4.

The laboratory will be able to provide different types of information at different times. The result of direct microscopy of specimens should be available within an hour, if necessary. Preliminary culture results with direct antibiotic sensitivity test results will usually be available at 18 to 24 hours after submission, with more definite information and further sensitivity test results at 48 hours. For nearly all specimens, the laboratory should be able to issue final reports including identification of pathogens and antimicrobial sensitivity results within 72 hours. Exceptions to this rule will include some blood cultures and all cultures for tubercle bacilli.

Serological work

Serological work is concerned with the patient's antibody responses to presumed microbial infection. The technique is a useful one but subject to severe limitations.

(1)   It is necessary to decide which infections may be relevant so that the patient's serum may be tested against the appropriate microbial antigens.

(2)   A single test is only very rarely of diagnostic value, at least two samples taken 10 to 14 days apart being required to assess changes in antibody levels.

(3)   Cross reactions of antibodies with several different, often unrelated, antigens are common, so that the results of tests may not be specific.

(4)   Antibody responses to 'irrelevant' antigens met in the past (anamnestic responses) may be evoked by current infections.

(5)   The evidence obtained by this approach is based on the assumption (usually correct) that the antibody response observed is evoked by tissue response to invading micro-organisms. This is, however, only an assumption, with the result that antibody tests are never as secure a means of establishing a diagnosis as is culture of the pathogen.

Serological test results must be interpreted discriminatingly by the clinician, in full knowledge of the clinical circumstances, if false conclusions are not to be drawn.

Under ideal circumstances, the laboratory receives two samples of clotted blood, taken one to two weeks apart, from a patient suspected of a particular infection: the first sample having been collected as soon as the clinician began investigations. The request form accompanying the samples should give enough information about the clinical problems of the patient to enable the laboratory staff to set up the tests requested by the clinician (when appropriate) and any others which may be helpful. At the same time, every effort should be made to isolate the pathogen thought to be causing the infection. If all goes well, it may then be possible to assess the cultural and serological findings together in the light of the patient's clinical state.

A case of enteric fever may provide an example of the correct approach. This septicaemic infection with *Salmonella typhi* (or with paratyphoid organisms) sometimes presents diagnostic problems. If *S. typhi* is recovered from the blood cultures of a patient with characteristic symptoms and signs, the patient is considered to have the disease. If blood cultures yield no growth, but the organism is recovered from the faeces, the patient may either have enteric fever or be an asymptomatic intestinal (biliary) carrier of *S. typhi* who now has an intercurrent febrile episode caused by something else. If the patient concurrently develops an antibody response to *S. typhi* which becomes more marked as he becomes more unwell and which diminishes as he recovers, then the antibody response is valuable evidence that the *S. typhi* is involved in causing his disease. The cultural evidence alone is insufficient, but the additional serological findings may substantiate the diagnosis. In a patient in whom all blood, faecal and urinary cultures are persistently negative for *S. typhi*, the antibody response may also be of some clinical value. If his Widal test shows a characteristic change in levels of antibody reacting with the antigens of *S. typhi* alone, this may support a diagnosis of current infection by the organism. If his serum shows changes in levels of antibody to antigens of *S. typhi* and to those of *S. paratyphi* A and *S. paratyphi* B, it may merely be showing an anamnestic response to antigens previously encountered by TAB immunization. The use of a battery of antigens in the test system reduces the chance of cross reactions being misinterpreted.

A single antibody reading in the Widal test in early infection is of no interpretive value: only changes in the test results as the disease develops offer any useful information. For this reason, laboratories often will not undertake such tests until they have two suitably timed specimens from the patient to examine. The results of serological tests may thus be delayed beyond the time when they may influence the management of an acutely ill patient.

Single specimens may be sufficient in diagnosing some infections (e.g. syphilis). However, even under such circumstances, repeated tests may still provide evidence of therapeutic response. Those requesting such tests must remember their non-specific nature and the possibility that the results given may relate to past, rather than present, infections. Serological tests must be interpreted in the light of the clinical findings: it is important to treat the patient and not the laboratory report.

Specimen collection

The clinician and the laboratory should collaborate to the greatest possible extent in order to provide the former with the maximum useful information obtainable by the latter. A number of things can be done to improve this collaboration which is, in practice, often far from ideal.

Specimen collection and transmission

Specimens should be collected at the clinically appropriate times. Those specimens which have little or no value (e.g. non-purulent sputum; sputum from patients receiving antibiotics; swabs from uninfected sites, and throat swabs from patients with unexplained fever and a normal throat) should not be collected at all and nor should specimens be collected 'out of time' (e.g. blood cultures from patients whose acute septicaemia was successfully treated 10 days before, or 'check' cultures of cerebrospinal fluid in recovered cases of meningitis). This will save the patient some discomfort and even risk, will save costs (an average specimen sent to my laboratory costs £4—£5) and will free the laboratory staff to concentrate on more useful specimens.

The correct specimen should be collected. For example, cervical swabs are more likely to be useful than vaginal swabs for the diagnosis of gonorrhoea in women, and stool should be collected rather than rectal swabs from those suspected of harbouring intestinal pathogens (there should not usually be much difficulty in producing appropriate material from patients with diarrhoea). When pus is available, several millilitres should be sent, not just a swab which has been dipped into it.

The collection of the specimen should be undertaken with appropriate care and not be entrusted to the unskilled. For example, high vaginal swabs should be collected under direct vision using a vaginal speculum, and throat swabs should be applied to both fauces using a spatula, again under direct vision.

Specimens should be collected into the appropriate, laboratory approved container which should be labelled with the patient's correct name and hospital number (if any); the name of the ward or department; the date and time of collection, and the nature of the specimen. Failure to do this wastes time and leads to many specimens being discarded. Swabs which may dry out should be placed in transport medium to prevent this. The container must be checked before despatch to ensure that the contents will not leak. Containers which arrive in the laboratory with biological materials on the outside are discarded to avoid risk to staff.

Once a specimen has been collected, it should be sent to the laboratory without delay. This will minimize the loss of delicate organisms through the drying out of the specimen and will also reduce the overgrowth of contaminating commensals. Routine specimens from inpatients should reach the laboratory early in the day.

When a request for investigation gives the impression of an ordered thought process on the part of the requesting doctor, the laboratory staff tend to respond by doing their utmost to help. It is almost impossible to maintain a high standard of laboratory work when numerous routine specimens are sent which seem to bear little relation to the patient's needs. Morale is especially affected when these arrive late in the day when the little remaining time (and any overtime) would be better spent on urgent investigations affecting the immediate management of the patient.

Information accompanying the specimen

Request forms should be completed by the investigating clinician or by others under his supervision and should always accompany the relevant specimen to the laboratory. The patient's name, age, sex and hospital number (if any); the name of the requesting doctor; the appropriate destination for the report, and the precise nature of the specimen should be (but often is not) entered legibly on every request form. The responsibility for ensuring that this is done lies with the requesting doctor. Serious errors can result from the neglect of this responsibility. For example, a patient was once nearly sent to a sanatorium because acid fast bacilli were found in sputum from another of the same name and initial who had been admitted to the same ward after the first patient's specimen had been forwarded. Neither form bore a hospital number; the name, Whelan, was not common, and the mistake was only discovered because the consultant thought the result very unlikely and heard about it before arrangements for transfer were complete.

A good specimen with an incomplete form is often processed because the laboratory staff do not wish to prejudice any contribution they may make to the patient's recovery. However, when a potentially dangerous microbe is isolated which may harm not only the patient but others in the ward, and there is no indication from which ward or department it came, the frustration of the laboratory staff attempting to notify the result can easily be imagined.

The exact nature of the investigation requested should be indicated and truthful reasons should be given for requesting it. If this means writing something indicative of desperation (e.g. 'Have tried everything else fruitlessly', or 'Help!') this is more likely to win the laboratory staff's sympathy and assistance than learned sounding dissimulation.

The laboratory may need supplementary information in order to do justice to the specimen. If the patient is receiving antibiotics this should be indicated and the drugs listed. If a wound swab is sent, information should be given as to the site of the lesion, how long it has been there, whether it is a 'clean' wound or a 'dirty' one, whether there is a surgical drain in position, and so on. Without such guidance, the laboratory will not be able to produce helpful reports. If a patient is being investigated for a fever, the laboratory should be told how long it has been present and whether non-standard techniques will be needed. Blood cultures are commonly discarded by the laboratory after 7 to 10 days if they yield no growth, but will be kept for much longer if infective endocarditis or brucellosis are suspected. Special cultures for actinomycosis or mycoplasmal infection will not be set up unless the laboratory staff are given enough information to think such diagnoses likely.

Any possible unusual risk to laboratory staff from handling the specimen should be indicated by marking the specimen and the form as high risk, and packing the specimen accordingly. The nature of the risk should be clearly stated. A blood culture request marked 'pyrexia of unknown origin' is not as helpful as one marked 'PUO from West Africa — possible Lassa fever'. People working in microbiology laboratories are not alarmist about their work, but they are aware of the marginal risks of infection which they run and so work in ways designed to minimize these risks. They are entitled to have their attention drawn to unusual risks as early as possible.

If an investigation is urgent, this should be indicated, with reasons; the clinician should make special arrangements with the laboratory, and should see that the specimen is delivered there urgently.

Investigation of infectious diseases

Most episodes of infectious disease, or of suspected infection, are straightforward and are easily diagnosed. A minority of patients present diagnostic problems of greater severity, some of which are never finally elucidated. The best results are achieved by carefully planned investigation, each set of procedures following upon the results of the last. This is preferable both to the blunderbuss approach of initiating all possible investigations at the same time (which is trying to the patient and to the laboratory staff, as well as being very expensive) and to the very common practice of thinking of new tests day by day in a disorganized fashion (resulting in waste of time in hospital and consequent waste of money; in accidental repetition of tests, and in failing to collect specimens which should be taken at a particular time).

It should be remembered that most of the diagnostic problems occurring in the field of infection, as in other areas of medical practice, are not unique, but are variations upon recurrent themes. The details will differ from patient to patient, but the approach to their investigation should be standard. The clinician should devise, for each standard clinical situation, a systematic programme of investigations which will lead him to a diagnosis in an ordered way with minimum distress to the patient, with minimum reasonable delay and with due economy. Such schemes of investigation should be recognized to be of local applicability only, since the patterns of infection seen vary from place to place and from time to time. Some such systems of investigation (so-called algorithms) have been published and are worth considering as a basis for one's own individual investigatory schemes.

By way of example of the general approach, I propose to discuss, in outline only, the investigation of unexplained fever (pyrexia of unknown origin, or PUO). This seems to present some of the most difficult diagnostic problems and is often inadequately investigated. It will be assumed that the history has produced no localizing symptoms, and that careful examination of the patient has shown no abnormality other than to confirm an elevated body temperature. Part of the investigation will be a daily physical examination of the patient to check that no new physical sign such as abdominal mass, spinal tenderness, neck stiffness, pleural effusion or any of myriad other possibilities has emerged. A careful record of the patient's temperature should also be kept, the thermometer readings being made by someone other than the patient in order to reduce the chance of being deceived by the occasional attention seeker who does not have a fever at all.

Right at the beginning of the investigation, the doctor should consider all of the clinical circumstances and ask himself whether there is any possibility of the disease being viral. If there is such a possibility, specimens for viral culture (see Chapter 3) should be collected at once and be sent immediately to the laboratory accompanied by an 'acute' sample of blood for viral serological examination. It is important to do this as early as possible in the patient's illness, and not to wait until many other investigations have drawn a blank. The reason for this is that while the causative virus may be present in large numbers just before and at the time of onset of a viral infection, these numbers usually fall off rapidly thereafter. If the virological cultures are not set up early, the opportunity for making the diagnosis may be missed.

Certain basic laboratory tests should be undertaken immediately in patients with PUO. These include routine haematological tests (haemoglobin, white cell total and differential count with examination of a film, and erythrocyte sedimentation test), chemical tests (plasma urea, bilirubin, alkaline phosphatase, transaminases, proteins and protein electrophoresis) and urine microscopy and culture. The haematological tests may give clues of many kinds.

(1) The haemoglobin level may be low as a result of anaemia related to infection or to leukaemia.

(2) The white cell count may be elevated because of infection (e.g. abscess formation) or because of leukaemia, or be decreased as a result of conditions such as lymphoma, myelosclerosis or infiltration of bone marrow by carcinomatous deposits.

(3) Abnormal cells may be seen, suggestive of infectious mononucleosis, other viral infections or leukaemia.

(4) The erythrocyte sedimentation rate may be normal (unusual in infectious diseases) or increased. If very much increased it may suggest longstanding pyogenic infection, carcinomatosis or myeloma.

The chemical tests may indicate uraemia, abnormalities of liver function, cellular breakdown or protein disorders. Urine microscopy and culture may show haematuria, pyuria or casts indicative of renal damage, or unsuspected urinary tract infection. 'Sterile pyuria' will alert the clinician to the possibility of renal tuberculosis.

At the same time as beginning these investigations, the doctor should be asking his patient (and himself) a series of questions which may lead to additional first stage investigations. Examples of relevant questions are given below.

(1) When were the symptoms first noted? Longstanding fever gives rise to thoughts of longstanding infections such as tuberculosis: recent onset of fever to more acute conditions.

(2) Is there any pattern in the occurrence of the fever indicating possible diagnoses such as malaria, lymphomas or enteric fever?

(3) How old is the patient? Different infections may have a different age incidence.

(4) Has the patient been in contact with anyone with an infectious disease?

(5) Does the patient's occupation or other activities give any clues (e.g. brucellosis in veterinary workers, leptospirosis in sewage workers, ornithosis in bird fanciers)?

(6) Has he dietary fads such as drinking unpasteurized milk?

(7) Has he been abroad recently, and if so where? This may give rise to suspicion of malaria, enteric fever, amoebiasis, giardiasis or a host of other conditions, depending on the details.

(8) What immunizations has he received? These may modify the clinical picture of conditions such as typhoid fever.

(9) Has he been taking any drugs, proprietary or pharmacopoeial? These may produce drug fever.

(10) What is his past medical history? The present episode may be a late consequence or a recrudescence of long forgotten disease.

(11) What pets does the patient have? They may have transmitted infection to the patient.

(12) Does the patient have hypersensitivity reactions such as eczema, asthma or angioneurotic oedema?

Each of these questions, and others, may give rise to clues worthy of investigation by appropriate further tests.

Assuming that the diagnosis has not already become clear, the next stage will be to set up blood cultures. These may point to diagnoses ranging from infective endocarditis, brucellosis or enteric fever to unrecognized abdominal abscesses or osteomyelitis. Under these circumstances, it is appropriate to collect three separate sets of blood samples, preferably taken when the patient is shown to be febrile. The diagnostic return on taking more than three sets is negligible. The laboratory should be informed that infective endocarditis and brucellosis are part of the differential diagnosis in order that the cultures be incubated for a long enough time. At the same time as the first blood sample is taken, some additional blood should always be collected to act as a serological baseline (the 'acute' specimen) for any antibody tests which may subsequently be needed. The laboratory should be asked to save the serum, and a note should be made in the patient's record that this has been done so that a second sample may be collected 10 to 14 days later for comparison.

At this point it should be remembered that infection is not the only cause of fever. In a large series of cases of PUO it was found that around half were caused by infections, and that smaller percentages were attributable to malignant disease (including lymphomas), collagen diseases, degenerative diseases, hypersensitivity reactions and the action of chemical agents including drugs. Consequently, while the first and second stage microbiological tests outlined above are proceeding, other investigations aimed at revealing hidden malignancy and other masses such as occult abscesses, collagen disorders and so on should be undertaken. Out of consideration for the patient, the microbiological and other tests should be grouped so as to minimize the number of venepunctures. For example, blood may be taken before radiological contrast medium is injected intravenously.

Only when the first and second stage investigations have failed to reveal a diagnosis, does it become reasonable to begin the more disagreeable or more esoteric tests. It is at this stage that antibody tests to every likely and unlikely cause of PUO (toxoplasmosis, histoplasmosis, brucellosis, aspergillosis, cytomegalovirus infection, etc.) should be considered. Now, too, it begins to be sensible to consider whether bone marrow biopsy or liver biopsy may yield diagnostic information not obtained from blood cultures. Eventually, in severe cases, exploratory surgery or therapeutic trial of antibiotics may be resorted to.

In practice, the investigation of PUO will be varied in the light of clues emerging as tests proceed. This outline is offered merely as a guide to investigational design, and as such, is also applicable in principle to the investigation of other infectious clinical conditions.

3

Viruses, fungi and parasites

There is, of course, little in common between these groups of organisms and they deserve individual attention. In the previous chapter I discussed the general properties of bacteria, the nature of bacterial infections and the laboratory methods used in their diagnosis. In this chapter I propose to follow a similar plan for the other main groups of medically important micro-organisms, which are brought together here for convenience.

The viruses

> So, naturalists observe, a flea
> Hath smaller fleas that on him prey;
> And these have smaller fleas to bite 'em,
> And so proceed ad infinitum.
>
> *On Poetry*, Jonathan Swift (1667—1745)

The viruses form a large group of infectious agents parasitizing other microbes, plants, animals and man. There is a wide variation in particle size, but the medically important viruses range from 20 to 300 nm in diameter. The genetic material of a virus is composed of RNA or DNA but, unlike that of a bacterium, never both. Organisms such as the Chlamydiae which, because of virus-like properties, used to be regarded as honorary viruses but which contain both nucleic acids, are

41

now recognized to be bacteria. Surrounding the central nucleic acid core there may be a layer of protein sub-units arranged either spirally (in which case the virus is said to show 'helical symmetry') or in an icosahedron ('cubic symmetry'). Some viruses are surrounded by an outer membrane containing lipids. Most such enveloped viruses can be inactivated by exposure to lipid solvents such as ether. Just as Table 1 set out a simple classification of the bacteria using only shape, Gram stain response and aerobic or anaerobic growth, so Table 2 offers a simple classification of the main groups of medically important viruses using only nucleic acid type, nature of symmetry and presence or absence of an outer membrane.

Table 2   Provisional classification of viruses pathogenic to man (after Andrewes and Pereira, 1972)

Nucleic acid	Symmetry	Presence of outer membrane	Viruses
RNA	cubical	−	Picornaviruses, Reoviruses
		+	Togaviruses
	helical	+	Orthomyxoviruses, Paramyxoviruses, Rhabdoviruses
	uncertain	+	Arenaviruses, Coronaviruses
DNA	cubical	−	Papovaviruses, Adenoviruses
		+	Herpesviruses
	uncertain	+	Poxviruses

Advances in our knowledge of the properties of viruses have followed closely upon the development of new technology. Two major characteristics of viruses are their inability to propagate themselves outside their living host cells, and their small size. Research on viruses was therefore severely hampered until the introduction of tissue culture and electron microscopy. Most of the work prior to this, was conducted using bacterial filtrates (containing 'filter passing viruses') which provided a means of assessing the size of the viral particles by grading the pore size of the filter used. Such filtrates could then only be examined by inoculation into living animals. Subsequently, it became possible to propagate viruses in fertile hens' eggs, and later still, in tissue cultures. The application of light microscopy to virology produced only modest results due to the limited resolution of optical microscopes. However, the technique was of some value in the recognition of individual particles (elementary bodies) of some of the larger viruses and of clumps (inclusion bodies) of others in infected cells. The introduction of electron microscopy made it possible for the detailed structure of virus particles to be seen for the first time.

I have avoided using the word 'organism' in relation to viruses because it is difficult to describe as a living creature a structure which is incapable of replicating itself without the agency of the genetic material of alien cells, and which is capable of renewed activity after crystallization of its nucleic acid. The role of viral nucleic acid in relation to host cells is analogous to the plastic instruction cards inserted into some modern washing machines which select the sequence of tasks to be fulfilled by the machine. The process is initiated by the attachment and absorption of a virus to its host cell. The specificity of the relationship between host and virus is determined by the outer layers of the virus, and a 'good fit' is required for successful host—virus attachment. Naked viral nucleic acid may have a much wider range of possible hosts than the intact virus, the outer layers of which are antigenic and provoke the immune response of the host. Once attached, the virus is either ingested by, or injects itself into, the host cell. A quiescent (eclipse) stage follows, during which infective virus cannot be retrieved from the host cell. At this stage the viral nucleic acid is subverting the host cell's enzymatic armoury, by use of modifications controlled by the host's DNA, to forge new viral components and to assemble them into new virus particles. When a sufficient number of such virions has been generated, they are released from the host cell either by extrusion or by lysis, and are free to find new host cells and to repeat the process.

Commonly, cells can be invaded successfully by only one type of virus at a time, the multiplication of the second being prevented either by 'interference' (mediated by 'interferon') or by direct blocking by the first. Upon occasion, however, two dissimilar viruses can co-exist in the same cell and, under specialized conditions, the host cell may generate 'recombinant' virions with some genetic characteristics of each invading virus.

As has already been noted (Chapter 2), some viruses may remain quiescent for lengthy periods. This is the case with those temperate bacteriophages which do not lyse their host cells. These 'phages reproduce at the same time as their host and are passed down from generation to generation of host cells. Such lysogenized viruses may be released spontaneously or be 'cured' from their host cells by exposure to chemicals such as dyes or to ultraviolet light. In some cases, virus nucleic acid may integrate with the host cell's genetic material and alter the characteristics of the host cell (lysogenic conversion). One example of this is the production, under the influence of a 'phage, of diphtheria toxin by strains of otherwise non-toxigenic *Corynebacterium diphtheriae*. Another example is the virulence factor for the intestinal tract of young animals which is conferred by other 'phages on some serotypes of *Escherichia coli*. The occasional role of 'phages in accidentally carrying plasmids mediating antibiotic resistance or other characteristics from one bacterial host to another (transduction) has been mentioned in Chapter 2.

Laboratory methods in clinical virology, as in clinical bacteriology, are based upon microscopy, culture, and serological techniques.

Direct light microscopy of clinical specimens has little to offer except in a limited range of circumstances (e.g. the presence of inclusion bodies, of elementary bodies, or of atypical mononuclear cells or 'virocytes' seen in the blood films of patients with some viral infections). However, the use of the light microscope in the examination of tissue cultures inoculated with material containing certain viruses is an important diagnostic technique (see below). The value of microscopy as a diagnostic procedure has been transformed by the advent of the electron microscope. Some electron photomicrographs of viruses from clinical specimens are shown in Figure 1. Electron microscopy of suitably collected material has permitted the rapid identification (within 2 hours) of viruses (e.g. varicella zoster, herpes, variola and its variants, and orf) collected from vesicular lesions. Electron microscopy for rotaviruses from stools takes only a little longer. This rapid identification of pathogens from clinical material is much faster than anything so far available in bacteriological diagnosis. Using the technique of immunofluorescence, similarly rapid viral diagnostic methods have been developed for the demonstration of infection with respiratory syncytial virus (RSV), a troublesome respiratory infection in children, sometimes giving rise to respiratory obstruction. Methods of immuno-electronmicroscopy capable of giving rapid diagnostic information are now being developed.

Special precautions must be taken by laboratory staff in handling

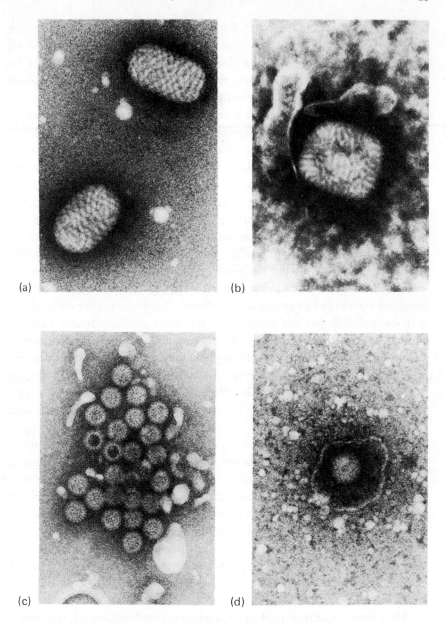

Figure 1: Electron photomicrographs of viruses from clinical specimens
(a) Orf (contagious pustular dermatitis), (b) Vaccinia, (c) Rotavirus,
(d) Varicella zoster. All magnifications 75 000 ×

material from vesicular lesions if there is any possibility that the lesion may be caused by smallpox, and such material should be examined only by designated smallpox diagnostic laboratories. This can be ensured only if clinicians inform their usual diagnostic laboratories of such a possibility before collecting the sample.

The second set of diagnostic techniques is based upon culture of viruses. This may be undertaken in laboratory animals, in fertile hens' eggs, or in tissue cultures. The inoculation of animals or eggs for viral diagnostic purposes has been largely supplanted by tissue culture techniques and is now used only for a relatively limited range of diagnostic procedures, such as the differentiation of Coxsackie viruses by injection into the brain of suckling mice. Tissue cultures are monolayer cultures, in bottles, of cell lines derived from mammalian or human tissues which retain their vitality and capacity to divide for lengthy periods provided they are bathed in a suitable fluid, containing nutrients and changed at appropriate intervals. These cell sheets can be infected by viruses from clinical material. As no particular cell culture will be suitable for the culture of all medically important viruses, clinical laboratories undertaking this work maintain several different cell lines to cover most of the likely possibilities. The cost of maintaining cell lines in good condition is high, and so those capable of growing some of the less common of the clinically important viruses are maintained only by specialized laboratories. Some therefore have to be sent on to such laboratories.

In order to obtain satisfactory results, the appropriate specimen must be taken early in the disease. It must be collected directly into a bottle of virus transport medium freshly thawed after removal from the freezer. Viral transport medium contains a mixture of antibiotics designed to kill contaminating bacteria. Cultures in transport medium must be sent rapidly to the laboratory where they will be refrigerated until they can be examined. The fullest possible information must be given as to the nature of the specimen, and of the underlying clinical problem, in order to permit the choice of appropriate cell lines for inoculation.

After tissue cultures have been inoculated and incubated, the multiplication of viruses may be observed by various means.

(1)   The production, in the cell sheet, of cytopathic effects visible

under the light microscope. These changes may be specific enough to permit provisional identification.

(2) The demonstration of viral antigens in the culture fluid.

(3) The demonstration of viruses by examination under the microscope of culture fluid or disrupted cellular material.

(4) The adsorption of red blood cells (haemadsorption) onto cell layers infected with myxoviruses, or paramyxoviruses.

(5) The use of immunofluorescence microscopy.

(6) The prevention of infection by other viruses (interference).

The many immunological techniques which are used to identify individual viruses will not be discussed here.

Specimens from sites readily colonized by viruses, sent to the laboratory for viral culture, should always be accompanied by the first of two samples of clotted blood (separated by an interval of 10 to 14 days). The serum from this blood can then be tested against any viruses isolated. The mere isolation of a virus from the throat, the nasopharynx or the stools of a patient does not necessarily invest that virus with pathogenic significance: it may be quite unrelated to the patient's illness. If, however, there is a change in the patient's antibody response to the cultured virus, and this change reflects the progress of the infection, that will be useful evidence of the rôle of the virus in causing the disease.

Such serological tests are more commonly used in trying to identify the cause of an infection when cultures have not been attempted, have failed to yield a virus, or are inappropriate. It is important to take two specimens of blood, 10 to 14 days apart, for purposes of comparison, since only changes in antibody level with time have any diagnostic value in most cases. The first of the samples should be collected as soon as the patient is seen, in order to give the best chance of demonstrating a diagnostic rise in antibody level as the infection progresses. The fullest possible clinical information should be given to the laboratory about the features of the disease including details of how long the patient has been unwell. This is necessary because, with many clinical syndromes, any one of a variety of viruses could be implicated and so the laboratory needs as much help as it can get to select an appropriate range of antigens to react against those antibodies possibly present in the patient's blood. As viral antigens are costly, well conducted laboratories will test only paired sera in this way: they will not normally examine a single blood sample. The numerous different serological techniques used in such tests will not be described here: interested readers will find details in textbooks on diagnostic methods in virology.

In the field of preventive medicine, virology laboratories are now expected to screen all pregnant women to establish whether they are immune to german measles (rubella). This is so that the non-immune can be offered immunization after delivery, so reducing the chances of producing rubella-affected babies in subsequent pregnancies. Any appreciable level of rubella antibodies in the blood ($\geq 1:16$) implies previous infection or immunization and hence immunity, whereas an absence of antibodies implies susceptibility to infection. In the course of such testing, some women are found to have very high levels of antibody to rubella. This may be insignificant or may reflect recent infection, potentially a hazard in the first months of pregnancy. Similarly, a woman in early pregnancy may have had contact with someone suffering from rubella, or she may fear that she has. Establishing whether a pregnant woman has, or has just had, rubella is important because it may be felt that the risk of producing a rubella-affected child justifies termination of pregnancy. It is also important that the results of the tests are produced quickly because termination of pregnancy becomes more difficult and more dangerous as the pregnancy proceeds. When the first blood sample tested does not show very high levels of antibody, comparison with a second sample collected 7 to 10 days later will either show a diagnostic rise, confirming current or very recent infection, or will show no change, indicating no risk. Appropriate decisions can then be taken. Alternatively, if very high antibody levels are found in the first sample, it may not subsequently be possible to show significant changes in level. Under such circumstances, the antibody activity can be shown by suitable techniques to be concentrated either in both IgM and IgG fractions of serum proteins or just in the IgG fraction. Such antibody fractionation may be performed on the first specimen to prevent delay. The presence of rubella IgM antibody is strongly suggestive of recent or current infection, and will give rise to appropriate gynaecological advice. The importance of good clinical information reaching the laboratory is obvious in this case: a history of actual or possible exposure of a pregnant woman to rubella should be clearly communicated, with the relevant dates, and the duration of pregnancy. A pregnant woman found to have rubella antibodies once need not be tested again in the same or in a later pregnancy even if she subsequently comes into contact with rubella.

Another problem causing much clinical anxiety and work for the laboratory is that of the patient with hepatitis. Hepatitis A and hepatitis B may both be spread by contact with infected blood, although the faecal—oral route of spread is usual with hepatitis A. Hepatitis B (serum hepatitis) is usually spread by blood or blood products although sexual spread, particularly in homosexuals, also occurs. There have been a number of outbreaks of hepatitis B in hospitals, attended by several deaths of patients and staff, and these have caused natural anxieties in medical and nursing staff and among organizations representing staff interests. Concurrently, tests have been developed enabling the surface antigen of hepatitis B (HBsAg), the so-called Australia antigen, to be detected in the blood of patients suffering from this disease. The antigen may be detectable in the blood of some patients for many months, or even years, after recovery from the infection.

Experience has shown the wisdom of testing all blood donors for the presence of HBsAg and of refusing to accept as donors those found to carry the antigen. Similarly, all patients admitted to renal dialysis units and the staff of such units should be clear of the antigen. Apart from these very specialized situations, the risks of transmission of hepatitis B between patients or between staff and patients are very small (assuming no sexual activity on the wards). It is, therefore, very ill-advised to undertake screening programmes or semi-systematic testing of patients or staff to identify those who are HBsAg positive, because it causes a group of near outcasts to be identified. There is always a temptation to stop a nurse, a surgeon or a dentist found to carry HBsAg from working. This is, in my opinion, quite unreasonable since the chance of such staff dripping their own blood into a patient's lesion cannot be great. It is better, therefore, not to test staff and so to spare them and their colleagues needless anxiety. I suspect that if HBsAg had not at first been called the Australia antigen it would have seemed less threatening and would have provoked less anxiety.

The fungi and yeasts

> Can any mortal mixture of earth's mould
> Breathe such divine enchanting ravishment?

> *Comus*. John Milton (1608–1674)

The members of this very large group of ubiquitous micro-organisms are distinctively plant-like, but lack chlorophyll. They cannot synthesize their own nutrients, and so derive their requirements from dead or living organic material. Fungi have rigid cell walls containing chitin, which give the organism its characteristic shape. The cells contain nuclei and often, granules of fat or starch. Single cells are characteristic of the yeasts, but many fungi have filamentous forms (hyphae) with many cells linked in ropes which may become densely packed and matted, giving rise to aggregations known as mycelia.

Although sexual reproduction can occur in some of the unicellular organisms, the usual means of propagation is asexual (e.g. by budding). The multicellular forms may reproduce asexually or sexually. The asexual mechanisms may be vegetative, by the accidental detachment of part of the mycelium and its regrowth in a new situation, or by a more deliberate method in which a variety of spore bearing structures are formed on specialized hyphae. The nomenclature and classification of these structures will not be dealt with here. As the sexual mechanisms of reproduction exemplified by the fungi scarcely concern the medically important members of the group, their description will also be omitted.

Yeasts and fungi can grow in a wide range of temperatures, but those involved in systemic infections of man normally grow at 37 °C, while those which cause superficial infections thrive at a lower temperature. Fungi may grow aerobically or anaerobically. The laboratory diagnosis of infection caused by yeasts and fungi is based on microscopy, culture, biochemical tests and serology.

Direct microscopy of smears from clinical specimens collected for bacteriological examination may reveal the presence of fungi or yeasts as single cells, budding forms, or hyphal forms. The presence of hyphae in a clinical specimen indicates a greater possibility of a pathogenic rôle for the organism. Sometimes the appearance of the organism is sufficiently characteristic to make the diagnosis, as when yeasts surrounded by large capsules are seen in the cerebrospinal fluid of a patient with meningitis caused by *Cryptococcus neoformans*. Skin scrapings, nail clippings or hair from patients with suspected superficial infections such as ringworm, may be examined microscopically, either directly, or after treatment with potassium hydroxide, in an attempt to recognize morphological characteristics typical of the dermatophytes *Microsporum* spp., *Trichophyton* spp., and *Epidermophyton floccosum*. If microscopy of specimen tissues is not successful, a microscopic examination of fungi cultured from such material will permit the recognition of distinctive features of each dermatophyte. In the case of systemic mycoses, the only specimen available may be tissue removed for biopsy or at postmortem examination. Histological examination of this tissue using suitable staining methods such as silver impregnation may lead to the diagnosis. Unless special staining methods are used, some systemic mycoses may be missed.

The mainstay of the laboratory diagnosis of most fungal infections is the culture of the causative agent. This is sometimes possible without the use of special cultural techniques since some organisms such as *Candida* spp. and *Aspergillus* spp. will grow on routine bacteriological culture media. However, most fungi require special media and even those which will grow on, say, blood agar, will grow more readily and quickly on specially developed media. Generally, fungi and yeasts grown in the laboratory are derived from sites with a rapidly proliferating bacterial flora which will overgrow them unless steps are taken to prevent this. Most fungal culture media used for primary isolation from clinical material contain antibiotics to prevent this bacterial overgrowth. Some of the ringworm fungi grow slowly, taking weeks to produce characteristic colonies. Such cultures must be kept moist and be kept sealed to prevent the seeding of the medium with contaminating fungi from the air. The appearance of colonies of fungi on standard culture media (colour, size and outline of colony, rate of growth, surface appearance) may help in identifying the organism concerned. Examination of the aerial structures of the colony by plate microscopy may be helpful, and microscopic examination of teased out, suitably stained (lactophenol blue) mycelial material may lead to the recognition of characteristic diagnostic

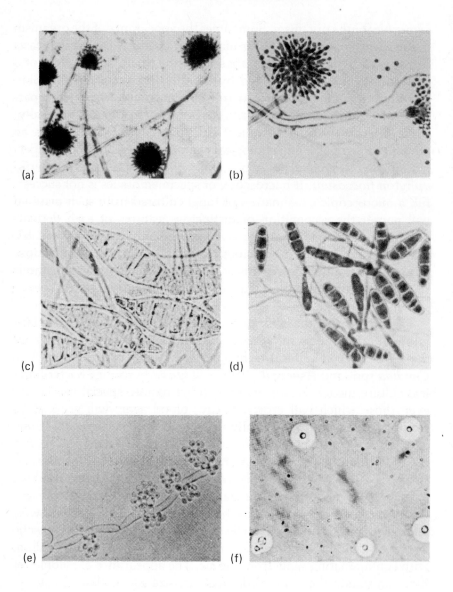

Figure 2: Photomicrographs of fungi and yeasts. (a) and (b) *Aspergillus* spp., (c) *Microsporum canis*, (d) *Epidermophyton floccosum*, (e) *Candida albicans*, (f) *Cryptococcus neoformans*. (Courtesy of The Upjohn Company, Kalamazoo, Michigan, publishers of a *Scope Monograph on Human Mycoses*)

features. The interested reader is referred to textbooks of mycology for more information. Some characteristic fungal structures are shown in Figure 2.

Biochemical tests on yeasts or fungi cultured in the laboratory play a much smaller part in their identification than do such tests on bacteria. Tests of utilization and fermentation of various carbohydrate substrates, with or without the production of gas, are performed in the identification of yeasts such as *Candida* spp., but few other chemical tests are used in differentiating fungi.

Serological procedures also play a smaller part in the diagnosis of fungal disease than in that of infections caused either by bacteria or by viruses. Serology may, however, be of great value in the diagnosis of systemic infections such as histoplasmosis and cryptococcosis, and may give some indirect evidence of tissue invasion in patients with candidiasis or aspergillosis. All the usual difficulties of interpretation of serological findings discussed in Chapter 2 apply to mycological serology.

The problems of interpretation of mycological observations in a clinical context may be considerable. Yeasts and fungi are plentiful in the environment, and so it may be difficult to decide whether any particular isolate is related to the patient's disease. In some situations, there will be little difficulty, as with the recovery of *Madurella mycetomi* from the depths of the lesion in a patient with Madura foot or of 'sulphur granules' from a patient with actinomycosis. Most clinical mycological situations are not so well defined. The problems are of two kinds: over diagnosis, and under diagnosis.

Over diagnosis happens particularly readily with the opportunistic organisms such as the yeasts and *Aspergillus* spp. The latter are very prevalent and may be found in the air, in soil and in dust. They are often found contaminating bacterial cultures, and are frequently present in diseased airways in man. Various clinical states may be associated with *Aspergillus* infection. These include rare skin infections; otitis externa usually associated with *A. niger*; aspergilloma of the paranasal sinuses generally caused by *A. flavus*, and invasive aspergillosis most often occurring in patients severely ill for other reasons. The main difficulties arise in the diagnosis of pulmonary aspergillosis because, while the isolated fungus may be associated with pulmonary disease, it may equally well be a contamin-

ant of the cultures, or a commensal in the patient. Pulmonary aspergillosis is generally caused by *A. fumigatus* and may present as a hypersensitivity reaction, as an aspergilloma or with invasive disease.
Hypersensitivity may take the form of asthmatic attacks, or a chronic
process (allergic bronchopulmonary aspergillosis) with fever,
pulmonary infiltration, eosinophilia, local and cutaneous immune
responses, and even bronchiectasis and localized peribronchial
invasion. Aspergilloma is a relatively benign condition in which pre-
existing cavities, left for instance by healed tuberculosis, are partially
or wholly filled with a ball of *A. fumigatus*. This usually causes little
trouble unless a pulmonary bloodvessel is incidentally eroded.
Invasive pulmonary disease caused by *A. fumigatus* is rare and occurs
in the immune-compromised host, generally proceeding rapidly to a
fatal conclusion with little evidence of local inflammatory response.

The assessment of patients with suspected pulmonary aspergillosis
is difficult and depends upon clinical and radiological findings as well
as upon laboratory methods. Antifungal drugs are often toxic and so it
is particularly important to treat the patient and not the pathology
report. Mere isolation of *A. fumigatus* from the sputum is not
sufficient for diagnosis. The demonstration of an antibody response is
common with aspergilloma but less frequent with hypersensitivity
reactions. The patient rarely develops a detectable antibody response
to systemic invasion by *A. fumigatus*. Precise diagnosis is important
because it will determine subsequent management of the patient:
inactivity in the commensal state; inactivity or resection of the lesion
in aspergilloma; steroid therapy possibly combined with imidazoles
for bronchopulmonary aspergillosis, and amphotericin B for invasive
aspergillosis.

The tendency to underestimate the significance of fungi is exemplified by an unfortunate patient seen in hospital some years ago. He had
an unexplained fever lasting many weeks during which the whole
gamut of clinical, radiological and laboratory investigations were
undertaken without result. He was given various courses of antibiotic
treatment, all to no avail, and he eventually died without anyone
having any idea why. His postmortem examination was well attended
and revealed massive fungal abscesses of brain, lungs, liver, spleen,
lymph glands and bone marrow. The pathologist performing the
autopsy was at a loss to know why such extensive fungal invasion had

not resulted in the isolation of the causative organism from blood cultures. Examination of the work records in the bacteriology laboratory showed that more than a dozen sets of blood cultures had been examined and that most of the bottles had been discarded after a few days' incubation because a yeast found growing in them was mistakenly assumed to be a contaminant. Good laboratory supervision is essential.

The choice of antifungal chemotherapy has widened considerably in recent years. There used to be few useful drugs available other than griseofulvin for ringworm, nystatin for yeast infections and the potentially nephrotoxic drug, amphotericin B, for systemic infections. More recently, 5-fluorocytosine and a whole new group of imidazoles (clotrimazole, miconazole, ketoconazole and econazole) have become available. In case of doubt, expert advice should be sought on drug choice and dosage. This may prevent further tragedies such as those reported by Symmers (1973) in which a series of patients with fungal infections were fatally under treated because their doctors were so concerned about the toxicity of amphotericin B that they did not give enough of this potentially life saving drug.

The protozoa and helminths

> While the angels, all pallid and wan
> Uprising, unveiling, affirm
> That the play is the tragedy, 'Man',
> And its hero the Conqueror Worm
>
> *The Conqueror Worm.* Edgar Allan Poe (1809—1849)

The organisms in these two groups are enormously varied. Although transmission is commonly direct from man to man in some, the majority require the intervention of an insect or other vector, and for a number of species there are important animal reservoirs of infection. Complicated life cycles involving two or more hosts and tenuous connecting links often make the chain of transmission extremely inefficient, so that hundreds of thousands of parasites die unfulfilled for every one completing a full life cycle and becoming capable of initiating the next. Nevertheless, aided by poor standards of sanitation and hygiene, the parasites are all too successful. They cause some of the most prevalent diseases in the world, and the consequences in terms of human misery and economic loss are enormous.

Some of the organisms concerned are, at one stage of their lives, so large that they scarcely fall within the remit of microbiology. The mature pork tape worm *Taenia solium* and the beef tape worm *Taenia saginata* may be several metres long and are easily seen with the naked eye. Common round worms (*Ascaris lumbricoides*), whip worms (*Trichuris trichiura*) and thread worms (*Enterobius vermicularis*), although much smaller than the tape worms, are all, at one stage of their careers, visible without a microscope. For the most part, however, the group is made up of organisms (including those named above) which are very small at the preliminary stages in their development, and which either remain minute in size throughout their cycle, or, despite having grown large at some stage, still require microscopic examination for final identification (such as the differentiation between *T. saginata* and *T. solium*).

Laboratory diagnosis rests upon microscopy, culture and serological methods. The most important of these is microscopy, which commonly involves the phase in the life cycle at which the parasite usually leaves the human host. It is not necessary to know in detail every phase of every cycle.

Examination of faeces for ova or cysts requires the use of appropriate concentration methods. If active trophozoites of *Entamoeba histolytica* are to be sought in material from patients with suspected amoebic dysentery, stool specimens must be examined in the laboratory while they are still quite fresh. In temperate climates this diagnosis is, sadly, not often entertained when there is no history of foreign travel, and the patient may suffer by being treated inappropriately for presumed ulcerative colitis when a simple stool examination or serological test would have given the correct diagnosis. Most experienced medical microbiologists have seen this diagnostic misfortune happen more than once, sometimes with quite disastrous results. The identification of ova or cysts in faeces is a skilled task, best undertaken by those with experience, because the differentiation between pathogenic organisms which may require eradicative chemotherapy (such as *Entamoeba histolytica*) and harmless organisms which should be left alone (such as *Entamoeba coli*) is crucial. Some organisms, such as *Schistosoma haematobium*, may be sought in the urine by microscopic examination.

The examination of suitably stained, thick and thin blood films for malarial parasites is an essential diagnostic investigation for any febrile patient in (or from) an area in which malaria is endemic. Usually it is not too difficult to see malarial parasites within red blood cells if they are there, but occasional patients present great difficulties in this regard. Experience is required to identify the particular stages of development which may be present, and still more expertise is needed to identify the infecting species (*Plasmodium vivax*, *P. malariae*, *P. falciparum* and *P. ovale*), a differentiation which may be crucial because it should be used to guide drug choice. In temperate climates, lives are lost every year because blood smears are not examined for malarial parasites, because the examination is inexpertly done, or because correct laboratory findings do not lead to appropriate drug selection. In case of doubt, expert advice should always be sought.

Microscopic examination of blood collected at night may reveal the presence of microfilariae (*Wucheria bancrofti* or *Brugia malayi*) which cause filariasis, while similar findings in blood collected by day may identify the eye worm *Loa loa*. *Onchocerca* spp. (the cause of river blindness) are found in skin snips.

Histological examination of tissues removed by biopsy, surgically, or at autopsy may reveal lesions recognized as being caused by the tape worm *Taenia solium*; encysted larvae of *Trichinella spiralis*; filarial granulation tissue; cysts of hydatid disease caused by *Echinococcus granulosus* or *E. multilocularis*; the lesions of schistosomiasis; amoebic liver abscesses; damage due to leishmaniasis; pulmonary infection caused by *Pneumocystis carinii*, and many other features of parasitic diseases. In temperate climates, experience of the histological features of many parasitic diseases is difficult to accumulate so that specialist opinions may need to be sought by those histopathologists who do not have a special interest in this field. Species identification can sometimes be made by immunofluorescence of paraffin sections.

Although cultural methods exist for the propagation of some protozoa in the laboratory, relatively little use is made of them in laboratory diagnosis. However, they are important for *Leishmania* spp. which are not always found by direct microscopy. Another exception in some laboratories is the use of culture media to increase the yield of *Trichomonas vaginalis* from vaginal swabs. However, opinions vary as to the value of such cultures, and many diagnostic laboratories do not use them, preferring to rely upon direct microscopy of vaginal smears. Culture is important for the preparation of antigens for laboratory use and for the testing of new drugs.

A variety of serological techniques have been developed to test the patient's antibody response to invading parasites. Some of these are not generally available because of difficulties in obtaining satisfactory material for the preparation of antigens. With others, notably the round worms (nematodes), the antigens are deplorably non-specific. In some diseases, more than one type of test is necessary to obtain a reliable conclusion. In spite of these problems and those connected with the interpretation of serological tests in general (see Chapter 2), serology may be the only practicable approach to diagnosis in an important range of diseases in which the parasite is frequently inaccessible to the microscope. These diseases include amoebic liver abscess, amoeboma, Chagas's disease, hydatid disease, cysticercosis and pneumocystosis. Test results for some of these can be up to 95% reliable. For other diseases, serology is used as an adjunct to diagnosis or as a test of cure. Skin tests are useful in some types of leishmaniasis, but serology is generally preferable when available. Both are important epidemiological tools.

No account has been given here of the life cycles of medically important parasites, of the control of their spread or of the treatment or prevention of parasitic diseases. The travels of some parasites from habitat to habitat and from host to host match some of the more improbable exploits of Odysseus, and are well worth the attention of romantically inclined readers. These (and others) are recommended to read textbooks and reviews on the subject.

4

Antibacterial drugs

Cur'd yesterday of my disease,
I died last night of my physician.

The Remedy Worse than the Disease, Matthew Prior (1664—1721)

The central question is: when to treat? The answer, as in other thera-peutic situations, is: when the expected benefits far outweigh the prob-able costs. Costs, in this context, are of several kinds:

(1) side effects suffered by treated patients;
(2) ecological damage tending to reduce the future effectiveness of the drug used (and possibly of others) and perhaps to increase the number of people infected, and
(3) financial expenditure.

Each of these limitations is sufficiently important to be individually considered.

Side effects of antibiotics

Side effects of antibiotics exercise important constraints on their use. On the one hand, the knowledge that serious problems may ensue from treatment should prevent the use of antimicrobial agents for trivial, self-limiting infections and for those in which their use is not proved to be beneficial. On the other hand, the possibility of doing harm should not cause appropriate treatment to be withheld from patients with serious infections. Minor infections such as those of the upper respiratory tract, boils and drained abscesses should generally not be treated with antibiotics. Lesions which may be bacterially *colonized* but are not *infected*, such as most weeping skin lesions, varicose ulcers and nappy rash should not be considered indications for chemotherapy either. This latter group should not even be investigated bacteriologically unless there is a clinical suspicion of active infection. Otherwise, there is the possibility that the laboratory will report the presence of the predictable coliform organisms together with their antibiotic sensitivities on the assumption that the clinician would not have requested the investigation without good reason. The clinician, in his turn, may then assume that the laboratory staff would not have reported the antibiotic sensitivities unless they had thought the bacteria to be pathogenic. This sort of clinico-pathological misunderstanding can generate needless prescription of antibiotics.

Information on the side effects of antimicrobial therapy will influence choice of treatment. It is desirable to know firstly, the type and severity of side effects to be expected when particular drugs are used and, secondly, the frequency with which side effects occur. The prescriber knows, for example, that about 5% of patients receiving oral ampicillin, amoxycillin or talampicillin will notice some bowel upset. This is an effect which, though common, is sufficiently mild not to deter the prescriber in most cases. On the other hand, clinicians are deterred from prescribing a 'dangerous' drug even if the severe side effect which they fear occurs rarely. An example of this is the irreversible bone marrow damage, culminating fatally, which occurs in one patient in about thirty thousand treated with chloramphenicol.

Doctors are often irrational about this. Chloramphenicol is now used for only very limited indications (*Haemophilus influenzae* meningitis, enteric fever) because of the fear of killing one in thirty thousand patients with this 'very dangerous' drug. The same clinicians would scarcely worry about using penicillins (with a death rate from anaphylaxis of approximately one in fifty thousand) or sulphonamides (with a death rate of approximately one in one hundred thousand from Stevens—Johnson syndrome) in the same way, because neither drug is considered dangerous. What is needed is a sense of proportion. All antibiotics are rather more dangerous than is commonly realized.

They should, therefore, be used less often but with more determination. A doctor considering whether to treat a particular patient should think about the realistic chances of doing harm and the type of damage which may ensue. If the patient has a minor, self-limiting infection, chemotherapy may achieve little. A fatal outcome of treatment under such circumstances is a catastrophe. If the infection is of greater severity, the choice of an appropriate antibiotic should scarcely be affected by the (remote) chance of fatal side effects.

Some drugs worry doctors more than others. Amphotericin B treatment has been described (Symmers, 1973) as giving rise to a phobia of such severity among clinicians as to result in patients dying of untreated or under treated fungal disease. The similar fear of chloramphenicol (a very potent and useful, but under used drug) has already been mentioned. In my current experience, I find clinicians to be worried about the use of gentamicin. This is a very useful, lifesaving drug which happens to give rise to vestibular damage if the patient is given too much. This should cause clinicians to avoid its use except for serious infection. When properly indicated, however, it should be given in quantities capable of eradicating the infection. Better an unsteady patient than a dead one! The laboratory should be able to undertake gentamicin assays to guide dosage so as to achieve only the desired effect. Incidentally, many of the patients now being given gentamicin in our hospitals would be better served if they were given chloramphenicol or co-trimoxazole instead.

Experienced doctors are aware that patients expect side effects from antibiotics and that they are very likely to attribute untoward events, including effects of their illness, to antibiotic use. In times such as these, when patients are more litigious than previously, clinicians would be wise to avoid antimicrobial therapy for marginal clinical or social indications.

Antibiotic resistance

Laboratory testing of bacteria for sensitivity to antimicrobial drugs may demonstrate predictable sensitivity at one end of the range (e.g. strains of *Streptococcus haemolyticus* (Group A) are virtually always sensitive to penicillin), and predictable resistance at the other (e.g. *Proteus mirabilis* strains are resistant to tetracycline, and the staphylococci are resistant to nalidixic acid). In between, are the far more numerous examples of bacteria for which the results of testing are not individually predictable. Occasionally a change in the predictable sensitivity of a species occurs. Recent examples are the occurrence of penicillin resistance in the gonococci and the identification of varying degrees of resistance to penicillin in pneumococci of different types from Papua New Guinea and South Africa.

When a new antibiotic is introduced, it is usual to find that most strains of a species are sensitive to it, but that as the years go by and the drug is more heavily used, more and more strains become resistant. This may happen as a result of:

(1) the stepwise accumulation of small degrees of resistance through minor bacterial mutations (as may occur during exposure to streptomycin);

(2) a single step bacterial mutation to massive resistance, although this is rare, or

(3) the transfer of genetic material mediating antibiotic resistance from one organism to another at bacterial 'mating' (conjugation), by the agency of bacterial viruses (transduction) or through other mechanisms of bacterial component swapping (transformation). Sometimes, the transferable bacterial genetic components mediating resistance, known as R factors, code for resistance to not only one antibiotic or group of antibiotics, but to several often unrelated drugs.

The spread of antibiotic resistance in bacterial populations carried by man is nearly always mediated by the elimination of sensitive strains and their replacement by resistant ones, as a result of antibiotic use. The greater the amount of antibiotic used, in general, the greater the prevalence of resistant strains. Antibiotic resistant bacteria generally, however, are somewhat less vigorous than their sensitive counterparts, so that if antibiotics are withdrawn from use, the resistant bacteria are often replaced by a sensitive flora.

This knowledge suggests that clinical bacteriology laboratories should keep records of the sensitivity to antimicrobial drugs of the pathogens which they isolate, since this will differ from place to place and from time to time. The information generated from such studies is of value in two ways: (1) as a guide to 'blind' treatment pending the results of laboratory tests and (2) as an indication of local accumulation of resistant bacteria, perhaps showing the need for a change in prescribing habits in order to restore the value of particular drugs.

Table 3 Proportions of all urinary pathogens fully sensitive to various antimicrobials 1971–78

A: General practice

Drug	Percentage of strains fully sensitive (Ranking)				
	1971 n = 433	1972 n = 418	1974 n = 585	1976 n = 681	1978 n = 606
Ampicillin/Amoxycillin	88.2 (4)	84.4 (6)	81.2 (7)	80.9 (7)	79.4 (7)
Cephalosporin	87.5 (5)	85.1 (4)	83.1 (6)	81.6 (6)	84.5 (6)
Colistin sulphamethate	85.0 (7)	82.3 (7)	87.9 (4)	85.0 (4)	90.3 (4)
Co-trimoxazole	96.6 (1)	96.4 (1)	93.2 (1)	96.7 (1)	97.0 (1)
Nalidixic acid	90.7 (3)	87.6 (3)	86.0 (5)	83.0 (5)	85.5 (5)
Nitrofurantoin	85.6 (6)	85.1 (4)	88.4 (3)	90.1 (3)	90.6 (3)
Sulphonamide	76.4 (8)	73.1 (8)	73.7 (8)	78.1 (8)	73.6 (9)
Tetracycline	72.5 (9)	69.6 (9)	73.6 (9)	74.5 (9)	75.7 (8)
Trimethoprim	94.0 (2)	94.4 (2)	89.5 (2)	92.7 (2)	90.9 (2)

B: Hospital practice

Drug	Percentage of strains fully sensitive (Ranking)				
	1971 n = 552	1972 n = 822	1974 n = 655	1976 n = 744	1978 n = 668
Ampicillin/Amoxycillin	66.1 (7)	64.2 (7)	61.2 (7)	53.7 (9)	51.2 (9)
Cephalosporin	69.9 (6)	68.1 (6)	63.2 (6)	57.2 (7)	58.2 (8)
Colistin sulphamethate	76.8 (4)	78.6 (4)	78.0 (2)	74.7 (4)	80.4 (3)
Co-trimoxazole	83.9 (2)	81.7 (2)	76.2 (3)	81.2 (1)	82.5 (2)
Nalidixic acid	84.8 (1)	82.6 (1)	80.6 (1)	75.3 (3)	85.5 (1)
Nitrofurantoin	70.3 (5)	71.5 (5)	72.7 (4)	73.2 (5)	74.4 (4)
Sulphonamide	61.9 (8)	62.2 (8)	57.4 (8)	58.9 (6)	58.5 (7)
Tetracycline	55.8 (9)	56.1 (9)	48.6 (9)	54.0 (8)	59.3 (6)
Trimethoprim	79.9 (3)	80.7 (3)	71.5 (5)	76.4 (2)	74.1 (5)

Table 3 presents observations on the antibiotic sensitivities of unselected urinary pathogens isolated in my own laboratory in the years 1971 to 1978. I shall use these data to illustrate a number of points as they arise. For the moment, let us consider the sensitivity of urinary pathogens to ampicillin and to the cephalosporins. Ampicillin and more recently the similar drugs amoxycillin and talampicillin, have been used very frequently because of their broad spectrum of activity and high level of safety. We can see from Table 3 that this heavy use of these drugs has resulted in decreasing sensitivity of urinary pathogens to them with the passage of time, both in general, and in hospital practice. The use of these drugs has also compromised the usefulness of the first generation of cephalosporins, resistance to which is mediated in the same way as resistance to ampicillin and the others. This is despite the fact that the cephalosporins have scarcely been used at all in and around the hospitals in which I work.

The ampicillins also give rise to problems in another way, because their use selects inherently ampicillin-resistant species such as *Klebsiella* spp. and *Pseudomonas aeruginosa* which tend to be resistant to many other antibiotics and therefore to give rise to infections which may be very difficult to treat. In a localized outbreak of infections caused by trimethoprim-resistant coliform bacilli (Grüneberg and Bendall, 1979) occurring in one of the hospitals in the University College Hospital Group some years ago, analysis showed that the predisposing factor was prior use of sulphonamide, co-trimoxazole or ampicillin, of which ampicillin was the most important. The clinical usefulness of co-trimoxazole in that hospital outbreak was restored by appropriate antibiotic restriction. A similar outbreak of hospital sepsis in a neurosurgical unit in Scotland was described by Price and Sleigh (1970), who managed to control it only by complete withdrawal of all antibiotics. They produced evidence that chemotherapy not only encouraged infections with antibiotic resistant organisms but that it also gave rise to an increased amount of infection.

It is important to realize that resistance to antibiotics rarely arises, during chemotherapy, among the bacterial population being treated. Thus, if amoxycillin is being used to treat an episode of urinary tract infection caused by a sensitive organism, the urinary pathogen will be exposed to high concentrations of the drug, and will usually be eliminated. Meanwhile, the bowel flora will also be exposed to the drug with the result that sensitive coliform bacilli will rapidly be replaced by resistant ones which may then give rise to reinfection of the urinary tract or to infection elsewhere. It is this unintended exposure of commensal bacteria to the selective pressures of chemotherapy which gives rise to the phenomenon of increasing bacterial resistance to antibiotics. If the problem continues to increase, we shall reach a situation in which the usefulness of the antibiotics is greatly restricted. It is, in consequence, the duty of prescribers to use no more antimicrobial chemotherapy than is essential. This means prescribing as few courses of antibiotics as possible, and ensuring that such courses are as short as possible. Treatment should be stopped when the infection is controlled. I have never understood the argument that treatment courses must be completed in order to prevent the emergence of resistance: once the drug has produced its desired effect, no further benefit can be expected, and it should be stopped for fear of selecting a resistant flora of commensal organisms.

Antibiotics are used in veterinary medicine and in agriculture to fatten livestock. It is very important that this should not jeopardize their successful use in man. Accordingly, the agricultural use of chemotherapy in feed supplementation has now (theoretically) been restricted, in Britain, to antimicrobials which are not used in human medicine (but see Chapter 9).

Cost of antibiotics

It is very difficult to obtain figures for expenditure on specific classes of drugs. However, it seems probable that expenditure on antibiotics is currently in the range £50—80 million per annum in the United Kingdom. In my own hospital, antibiotics account for approximately 1% of total expenditure and about 20% of drug costs. Spending of such magnitude becomes a matter of interest to administrators and politicians. Criticism is easily forestalled if antibiotics are used in such a way as to achieve good value for money, but this is often not the case.

The first example of financial cost which I wish to use is that of treating urinary tract infection (UTI). In general practice, it is almost impossible to demonstrate a better cure rate for UTI with any one of the usual drugs than with another. Other considerations, such as route of administration, side effects and cost, therefore become important in selecting a 'urinary' antibiotic. The cost of five days' treatment in standard dosage with some of these drugs is shown in Table 4. While these costs are simply those quoted in the University College Hospital at the time of writing and have no general validity, they will serve as a basis for comparison. Clearly, it is possible to achieve the same anti-microbial effect at widely different cost. In many cases, it will be appropriate to use cheaper rather than more costly drugs, but occasionally there will be good clinical reasons to prefer the more expensive preparation (see Chapters 5 and 6).

Table 4

Drug	Cost (£)
Amoxycillin	1.60
Cephalexin	1.60
Co-trimoxazole	1.26
Nalidixic acid	3.54
Nitrofurantoin	0.06
Oxytetracycline	0.13
Sulphadimidine	0.12

My second example is in the field of acute, undifferentiated chest infection. Again, any of a number of drugs will produce a similar clinical cure rate. The prices listed in Table 5 are the University College Hospital costs, at the time of writing, for 5 days' treatment in standard dosage.

Table 5

Drug	Cost (£)
Amoxycillin	1.60
Cephalosporin	1.60
Co-trimoxazole	1.26
Oxytetracycline	0.13

In this case, not only are there wide disparities in cost between these drugs, suggesting that the use of some of them is luxurious, but also it has been claimed (Howie, J. G. R. and Hutchison, K. R., 1978) that the justification for using any antibiotic in this kind of infection is slight, since a similar result would be achieved without chemotherapy.

One should not make too much of this general argument, but it should be accepted that what is spent on drugs cannot be spent on other, perhaps more important things. Clearly, when an expensive antibiotic is clinically appropriate, it should be used. In the generality of cases, however, drug choice should be influenced by the need for economy. It is surprising how often it is true that the cheaper drug constitutes the better clinical choice.

Having considered the three general constraints on antibiotic choice (safety, ecological background and cost), I propose to turn to a number of other topics concerned with antimicrobial chemotherapy.

The use of the laboratory

It is assumed that clinicians understand the importance of despatching suitable diagnostic specimens to the laboratory before starting antibiotic treatment. Failure to do this leads to decisions being made entirely on acumen (guesswork). This is sometimes necessary, as when no specimen can be collected or when the results of investigations cannot be awaited, but the limitations of this approach are obvious. Even under these circumstances, the laboratory should be able to help to determine the most appropriate choice of drug on a 'best guess' basis.

The results, presented in Table 3, of tests on all urinary pathogens in my laboratory in recent years, enable the laboratory staff to indicate the chances of an untested urinary pathogen being sensitive to any of the likely choices of drug. By this means it is possible to produce a ranking from best guess to worst guess as shown in Table 6.

There has been very little change at the top of this table in the years from 1971 to 1979. Co-trimoxazole has covered the widest, and tri-

Table 6 Ranking of various antimicrobial agents in UTI in general practice and hospital practice, 1979 (Percentage of strains fully sensitive)

General practice		Hospital practice	
1. Co-trimoxazole	(96.8%)	1. Co-trimoxazole	(80.8%)
2. Trimethoprim	(91.3%)	2. Nalidixic acid	(80.6%)
3. Colistin sulphamethate	(89.9%)	3. Colistin sulphamethate	(77.9%)
4. Nitrofurantoin	(89.5%)	4. Nitrofurantoin	(72.4%)
5. Nalidixic acid	(87.2%)	5. Trimethoprim	(69.8%)
6. Cephalosporins	(84.6%)	6. Cephalosporins	(60.5%)
7. Ampicillin/Amoxycillin	(72.9%)	7. Tetracyclines	(59.0%)
8. Tetracyclines	(71.4%)	8. Sulphonamides	(58.6%)
9. Sulphonamides	(69.5%)	9. Ampicillin/Amoxycillin	(54.6%)

methoprim the second widest, spectrum of urinary pathogens in general practice in every year. In hospital practice, co-trimoxazole and nalidixic acid have in turn shared the top position. It is noticeable that ampicillin/amoxycillin and the first generation cephalosporins have settled at the bottom of the table. (The choice of drugs for the treatment of UTI is discussed in Chapters 5 and 6.)

In most cases, proper samples can be sent to the laboratory for culture and for sensitivity testing of any organisms isolated, and the results will usually be available within 24 or 48 hours. This means that treatment can be adjusted promptly in the light of the laboratory findings.

The basis of most routine sensitivity testing methods is the exposure of a suitable inoculum of bacteria growing on a solid agar medium to antibiotic diffusing from an antibiotic-impregnated disk or strip. The size of the zone of inhibition of bacterial growth is measured and compared with suitable controls. This enables the test organism to be classified as sensitive, moderately sensitive or resistant to the antibiotic in question. The test is so conducted that the results give a general guide to likely treatment outcome. 'Sensitive' means that, in general, if the antibiotic is given in usual dosage it will be likely to eradicate the organism. 'Moderately sensitive' means that the standard dosage will not usually result in cure, but that a higher dosage may be effective. 'Resistant' means that use of the antibiotic would not be expected to eliminate the organism.

Much misunderstanding of sensitivity reports occurs because clinicians do not realize the limitations of the technique used. The laboratory may, of course, get the result of the test wrong for various technical reasons to do with the density of the inoculum, the suitability of the media, the adequacy of the controls, and so on; or because of transcription errors. Usually, however, the results reported by the laboratory are a correct statement of the effect of the antibiotics on the test organism *in vitro*. This does not, of course, always correspond precisely to what happens in the patient.

Sometimes a 'sensitive' organism is not eradicated from the patient by use of the appropriate drug. There are several reasons why this may happen.

(1)   An irrelevant organism may have been tested due, for example, to the overgrowth of contaminating organisms from

the mouth in a sputum sample delayed in transit to the laboratory.

(2) The antibiotic may not be absorbed properly and so not achieve adequate blood levels, as, for example, with the chelation of tetracyclines by milk products in the intestine.

(3) The antibiotic may not diffuse satisfactorily to the site of the infection, as in osteomyelitis or lung abscess.

(4) The presence of foreign matter, as in war injuries, may provide an impenetrable nidus in which bacteria may survive despite the production of otherwise adequate antibiotic concentrations.

(5) The original organism may be eradicated only to be replaced by another, so that the doctor may detect no clinical change.

(6) There may be other, unsuspected, pathogens present.

The opposite situation may also occur: an organism reported as 'resistant' being apparently eradicated by use of the inappropriate drug. In this case, the patient may not actually have been infected in the first place. A single urinary bacterial count of more than 100,000 organisms/ml, for example, will be confirmed in only 80% of cases when a second sample is examined. If only one sample is examined from patients thought to have urinary tract infection, UTI will be over-diagnosed accordingly and some of the non-infected symptomatic patients will have unexpected therapeutic success ('miracle cures'). Similarly, many infections recover without treatment, with the result that antibiotics are sometimes credited with clinical improvements for which they are not responsible.

Despite these various difficulties, it should be expected that the laboratory will produce antibiotic sensitivity results from which accurate predictions of the outcome of treatment can be made. Clinicians who are not convinced that this is so, should discuss their problems with senior laboratory staff in an attempt to clarify matters, rather than ignore the laboratory reports.

Monitoring treatment

In specialized situations, more detailed laboratory investigations will be required. There are, for example, two problems to be avoided during the use of the aminoglycoside, gentamicin: that of under treatment and that of over treatment. Antibiotic assays are therefore required to guide the administration of the drug. Under treatment can be avoided, theoretically, by measuring peak serum gentamicin levels to make sure that they are adequate. (The problem here lies in knowing when the peak level can be expected.) Over treatment is avoided by making sure that the smallest amount of gentamicin remaining in the blood, the so-called trough level just before the next dose is given, is not too high. The trough level will also indicate whether adequate treatment has been given. Failure to monitor serum gentamicin levels during treatment lasting for more than, say, 48 hours, is negligent. When assays are needed, there should be direct contact with the laboratory staff regarding time of collection of samples, and the clinician should mention any other antibiotics being given, since these may interfere with bioassay techniques.

Sometimes, it is appropriate to measure concentrations of other antibiotics: the concentration of penicillin in pleural fluid in cases of empyema, for instance. In cases of infective endocarditis the laboratory has a particularly important job to do. It should try to provide guidance about whether one antibiotic or a combination of two should be used; it should try to suggest which combination of antibiotics may be appropriate by testing pairs of drugs against the causative organism *in vitro*; it should measure the minimum bactericidal concentration (MBC) of the antibiotics used for the pathogenic organism, and it should back-titrate the antibiotic in the patient's serum to establish by how much the MBC is being exceeded during treatment. Failure to do this may result in under treatment of the endocarditis with subsequent relapse.

In all of these situations, the best results for the patient are achieved by close liaison between the clinician and the laboratory staff. The more contact there is at an early stage in the patient's illness, the better the outcome is likely to be. It is a nuisance for the clinical staff to have to provide information on bacteriology request forms, but without it the laboratory can provide only a very incomplete service. The type of specimen should be clearly described; the date and time of collection should be given; the names of *all* antibiotics being used should be specified (preferably with dosages), and any special clinical features such as pregnancy, renal failure or penicillin hypersensitivity should be mentioned. It is not sufficient to write 'wound swab' on a request form. In completing the form, the type of wound and its site and degree of contamination (if any) should be mentioned, and whether there is a drain or a prosthesis or other special feature should be indicated. Such information enables the laboratory staff to do a useful job and to provide the clinician with maximum support.

Specimens (of whatever kind) should reach the laboratory as quickly as possible in order to minimize delay, and to prevent the death of some organisms and the overgrowth of others.

Bactericidal or bacteristatic antibiotics?

Antibiotics are somewhat arbitrarily divided, on the basis of their *in vitro* properties, into two groups, the bactericidal and the bacteristatic. The distinction is not precise since high concentrations of bacteristatic drugs may be bactericidal and lower concentrations of bactericidal agents may be bacteristatic.

There is a widespread belief among clinicians, pandered to by representatives of some commercial interests, that bactericidal drugs are preferable to bacteristatic drugs.

This is unquestionably true in one clinical situation, that of infective endocarditis. In this disease, antibiotic penetration into infected vegetations on the heart valves is so poor, and there is so little tissue response in the form of phagocytosis or antibody action, to bacterial invasion, that failure of the antibiotic to kill the organisms outright will result in relapse after chemotherapy is stopped. This situation requires the use of bactericidal drugs.

It is sometimes suggested that infections in patients with granulocytopenia should be treated with bactericidal rather than bacteristatic drugs, but I find the evidence for this unimpressive. In all other clinical situations, it is unimportant whether the drug given is bactericidal or bacteristatic. Even in severe infections bacteristatic agents may suffice. In meningitis, for example, the bacteristatic agents chloramphenicol or sulphonamide are often used as drugs of choice.

Other severe infections may be treated with bactericidal drugs (pneumococcal pneumonia with penicillin, and acute pyelonephritis with ampicillin/amoxycillin, for instance) but the choice is not made on this basis. Representatives of drug manufacturers claiming that the bactericidal properties of their product confer advantages should be asked for clinical proof of this.

Antibiotic combinations

Antibiotics may be combined for several reasons: to cover all likely pathogens when the infecting organism is unknown; in an attempt to achieve synergism; in order to reduce the dosage of potentially toxic drugs; to prevent the emergence of bacterial resistance to the drugs given, or in the treatment of mixed infections.

The clinician is commonly faced with the problem of treating an ill, apparently infected patient in whom the nature of the infecting organism can only be guessed. The difficulty of finding a suitable antibiotic or antibiotic combination may be considerable. If the site of infection is known, this difficulty may be lessened. Gut-associated sepsis and gynaecological sepsis are both likely to involve aerobic and anaerobic organisms, both Gram-positive and Gram-negative. Penicillin + gentamicin + metronidazole, or clindamycin + gentamicin are possible antibiotic combinations for use in these cases. Similar mixtures are often used in the febrile (presumed infected) immunosuppressed patient. In my opinion such mixtures of antibiotics are used too much. They give rise to problems through their side effects; they often achieve little for the patient, and there is nothing more potent left in reserve if the patient's condition deteriorates. There really is no satisfactory antibiotic combination which will cover every type of organism reliably. I would prefer to see such combinations used only very briefly and only in support of other, non-antibiotic measures such as drainage of abdominal pus. The present, slightly casual use of antibiotic mixtures is to be deprecated. In my opinion, many patients would be as well treated if given only chloramphenicol or co-trimoxazole in the first instance.

The search for synergism between combinations of antimicrobial drugs has occupied a whole generation of clinical microbiologists in a way reminiscent of the alchemists' search for a means of turning base metals into gold. There are very few clinical situations in which there is good evidence of synergy. Sometimes a combination of two antibiotics which is synergistic against one strain is antagonistic when used against another. This means that rather than assuming synergism to be the likely effect, any proposed combination should be tested against the pathogen *in vitro* before use. The very word 'synergism' is of uncertain meaning except in a purely formal sense, and it is often wrongly used to describe 'additional' effects which could be obtained equally as well by giving more of one drug as by adding a second.

Reducing the dosage of toxic drugs by combining them is sometimes appropriate. An example is the combination of the nephrotoxic drug amphotericin B with 5-fluorocytosine in the treatment of sepsis caused by *Candida* spp.

Combination of drugs is often practised with the aim of preventing the emergence of resistant bacteria. This is the rationale behind combined chemotherapy of tuberculosis. The experimental and clinical evidence for the validity of this approach in non-tuberculous infections is, however, rather sketchy. It is most commonly advocated to 'protect' those antibiotics to which, when used alone, resistance emerges rapidly (e.g. rifampicin, fusidic acid).

The treatment of mixed infections with combined drugs gives rise to some of the worst abuses of this technique. Sometimes, infections occur with two or more equally sinister pathogens which should be treated together. The presence of both *Streptococcus haemolyticus* (Group A) and *Staphylococcus aureus* in a laceration of the hand, for example, might well justify the simultaneous use of flucloxacillin and penicillin. More commonly, however, a lesion yields a mixed growth of organisms containing one prime pathogen and a variety of other organisms of less significance. It is usually better under such circumstances, to try and eradicate the main threat with a single drug and then to reassess, rather than to try and hit everything by employing blunderbuss therapy. Many of the organisms isolated are probably relatively harmless commensals rather than pathogens.

The only combined preparation of antimicrobials on the market for general use at present is co-trimoxazole, a fixed ratio combination of sulphamethoxazole and trimethoprim. It was marketed in 1968 with the claim that its sequential blockade of two steps in bacterial folate metabolism gave it unique advantages; that the two components are synergistic; that it is bactericidal; that the combination delays the emergence of bacterial resistance, and that it has a very wide spectrum of antibacterial activity. Some now question the claimed advantages of sequential blockade; whether the drug is bactericidal seems to depend on the medium in which it is tested, and nobody really knows whether it does prevent the emergence of bacterial resistance. Nonetheless, it has established itself as a very valuable drug with a wide antibacterial spectrum; there has been little increase, generally, in resistance to its components among pathogens (see Table 3); it has an enviable record of safety, and there is evidence of synergy, as usually defined. This synergy is of value in the treatment of gonorrhoea and of some sulphonamide-resistant infections. The drug also has the advantage of suppressing the aerobic bowel flora, and so constitutes an excellent prophylaxis of infection in patients liable to reinfection of the urinary tract or in neutropenic patients at risk of intercurrent infection. Some, but not all, of these effects might be achieved by the use of trimethoprim alone, but critical comparative studies are lacking (Grüneberg, R. N., 1979).

Prophylactic chemotherapy

Early hopes that antibiotics could be used extensively to prevent infection in susceptible patients have largely been dashed, and the problem is seen to be much more complicated than was at first thought.

In general, the conditions under which prophylaxis can be expected to work are:

(1) the infection which is to be prevented is caused by one bacterial species or, at worst, by only a very few species;

(2) the causative organisms are always or nearly always sensitive to the drug to be used;

(3) the drug can be delivered in sufficient concentration to the likely site of infection; and

(4) use of the antibiotic does not induce bacterial resistance.

The drug should also be acceptable to the patient, safe and cheap. There are very few clinical situations which meet these requirements.

An example of prophylaxis that does work, is the use of penicillin to prevent recurrences of rheumatic fever in those with existing rheumatic heart disease. In this case, the disease is related to a single organism, *Streptococcus haemolyticus* (Group A) which is uniformly sensitive to penicillin. The use of the drug protects against infection and does not generate resistant strains of this organism. Other examples include the prevention of tetanus following penetrating agricultural or war injuries, by the use of penicillin, to which *Clostridium tetani* is always sensitive; the prevention of malaria, and the use of penicillin to prevent postoperative gas gangrene in patients suffering leg amputations for inadequate vascular supply. The use of prophylactic chemotherapy to cover dental manipulations in patients with damaged heart valves, with the aim of preventing infective endocarditis, has been well reviewed by Shanson (1980).

When ill-advised prophylaxis is attempted and the requirements for success listed above are not fulfilled, various consequences ensue.

(1) The infections are not prevented, 'breakthrough' infections invariably being caused by organisms which are resistant to the drug used and sometimes to other drugs as well.

(2) Antibiotic resistance becomes endemic in the bacterial population carried by patients in the unit concerned.

(3) Antibiotic use goes up alarmingly: if the target infection occurs normally in 10% of a group of patients, the use of antibiotic prophylaxis involving treatment of 100% of the population means a tenfold increase in antibiotic use over a policy of treating only the infected, whence

(4) The patients suffer ten times the number of side effects, and

(5) Costs increase by a factor of ten.

Clearly, there is no justification for attempting prophylaxis unless there is convincing proof that it will work (or unless a scientific study of its efficacy is being conducted) and that the infection which it is hoped to prevent is severe enough to warrant this sort of treatment.

In many of the clinical situations in which prophylactic chemotherapy is tried, it is doomed to failure. This is because many of the different organisms present may be pathogenic and because their antibiotic sensitivities are not predictable. Thus, the attempt to prevent postoperative chest infection by prophylactic chemotherapy does not work, and nor do similar attempts to prevent many forms of surgical sepsis. In some surgical situations, however, antibiotics instilled into the wound seem to reduce the number of episodes of postoperative sepsis, although not to prevent it entirely. It is not easy to make a definite statement about this in relation to sepsis following intestinal surgery because of the heated debate which is currently being conducted in the professional press by proponents of various antibiotic regimens. It seems unlikely to me that many of these antibiotic protocols are much more effective than the instillation into the wound, at operation, of povidone iodine (Stokes *et al.*, 1977). Povidone iodine is active against all bacteria, does not generate bacterial resistance, is harmless to the patient and is inexpensive.

In the light of the above discussion, I believe that clinicians should not use prophylactic antibiotics unless they can provide proof that such treatment will be effective. The onus of proof must be on the user.

Administration of antibiotics

Since detailed information is available from many sources I shall make some general points only.

No antibiotic should be given for longer than is clinically necessary. Unfortunately proof of the optimum time for treatment is, in most cases, lacking and when in doubt, clinicians tend to prolong treatment for fear of relapse. The serious hazards of interfering with the patient's commensal organisms and of increasing the spread of resistant bacteria among those treated for long periods have only gradually become apparent, but judging the correct time at which to stop treatment is almost as important as knowing when it should be started. The following are good reasons for stopping treatment:

(1) 48 hours without symptoms in simple infections such as uncomplicated urinary tract infections or acute bronchitis.

(2) Laboratory or other evidence which satisfies the clinician that the diagnosis of infection was mistaken or that the pathogen is resistant to the drug given. On no account should the 'course of treatment' be completed in these circumstances.

When there is a free choice, oral treatment should be preferred to parenteral routes. In parenteral chemotherapy, intramuscular injection is preferable to the intravenous route because high blood levels are sustained over a longer period. Intravenous treatment should, however, be used if the patient is shocked, in order to obtain adequate blood levels in the first hours of treatment. It is also sometimes necessary when very large quantities of drug must be given, as with carbenicillin. In this case, bolus injection or gradual infusion should be used. Antibiotic should not be added to the contents of an intravenous infusion bottle because it may be inactivated before it reaches the patient. However, it is considerate to inject antibiotics which may be painful when given intramuscularly, into the tubing of an intravenous drip, if this is already in use for some other reason. Intravenous drips should never be set up or maintained merely to administer antibiotics except in the special situation of drugs like carbenicillin, the volume of which makes this inevitable, or vancomycin which is too irritant to be given intramuscularly.

With most infections (or suspected infections), chemotherapy should be reviewed after 48 hours and stopped or changed if there is no obvious clinical benefit after 72 hours. Fever is not always caused by sepsis and may, indeed, be caused by antibiotics. 'Drug fever' is most commonly associated with the use of sulphonamides or penicillins. 'Blind' treatment, started after due consideration of the circumstances, should not be changed for at least 72 hours unless there is good reason to do so. Improvement in correctly treated enteric fever is not normally seen until at least the third day.

The frequency of dosing with antibiotics should be related to the halflife of the drug. This often means that there is an important distinction to be made between administration 'at 6-hourly intervals' and 'four times a day'.

The object of antibiotic treatment should be to attain, at the site of infection and for as much of the time as possible, a concentration of antibiotic greater than its minimum inhibitory concentration (MIC) for the pathogen. It is not usually useful to achieve many times this concentration. An exception to this rule is found in the treatment of infective endocarditis when an attempt should be made to obtain 5 to 10 times (but not more) the MIC of the drug for the pathogen in the blood. High dosage may also be used in the treatment of infections in sites with poor blood supply. This will provide very high blood levels of the antibiotic resulting, it is hoped, in adequate concentrations at the site of the infection. This approach may be used in empyema, lung abscess or osteomyelitis.

With many infections, chemotherapy may only be a part, even a relatively unimportant part, of the total treatment. Often drainage of a wound, the removal of a foreign body from it, or 'tipping and clapping' of an infected chest, are much more important than the use of drugs. Miracles should not be expected of the antibiotics, but much can be achieved by their intelligent use in combination with other forms of treatment.

Antibiotic prescribing policies

Antibiotic chemotherapy invites external intervention more than any other area of medical treatment. This is because the choice of antibiotics is so large and so constantly changing that it is difficult for clinicians to use them to their best effect; because their use leads to an accumulation of resistances; and because they are costly. Moreover, another group of specialists, the medical microbiologists, are likely to be in a position to help their colleagues since, while they must study the effects of these drugs, unlike the clinicians, they can afford to neglect advances in drug therapy of non-infective disease.

Antibiotic policies devised for the guidance of clinicians have three objectives, as follows:

Aim (1): To achieve the best choice of drug for the patient

The wellbeing of the patient must always be the overriding aim of treatment. The difficulty lies in making a sensible choice among the various possibilities. Clinicians are usually badly informed about antibiotics and get a great deal of confusing and biased guidance from the pharmaceutical industry. It is difficult enough for an 'expert' to assess the claims made for the many new products as they are released, but almost impossible for busy clinicians. Clearly, there is scope for those with a special interest to guide their colleagues. This can be done by sending out informative circulars or, more directly, by seeing the patients and offering specific guidance to the clinician. The advice given will be concerned with choice of drugs, dosage, route and frequency of administration, drug interactions, possible side effects and so forth. This approach is not acceptable unless the microbiologist, having seen the patient, reviews the circumstances and commits himself in writing. If the clinician then takes the advice he does so on the basis of shared responsibility.

As I have already indicated, two types of problem arise: under treatment and over treatment. The former is not very common but is exemplified by the clinical anxieties associated with the use of gentamicin described earlier in this chapter. The microbiologist's rôle here is to help the clinician by restoring a sense of proportion to the consideration of risks and benefits. His advice will be to treat serious infections seriously, and to be prepared to accept a price in possible side effects in return for the survival of the patient.

Overtreatment is more frequent. Either a sledgehammer is used to crack a nut, or an antibiotic is used when none is needed. Good prescribing in antimicrobial chemotherapy, as in other spheres, relies upon the principle of economy of effort: no more treatment should be given than is strictly necessary. The most serious problem is the use of antibiotics when none are needed. This ranges from the widespread abuse of antimicrobial prophylaxis, already discussed, to the vigorous treatment of minor, self-limiting infection. When the possible benefits from treatment are slight, antibiotics should not be used. The most frequent piece of advice on chemotherapy which I give to my clinical colleagues when I see their patients, is to stop all antibiotics.

When it is clear that the patient is infected but before the pathogen and its sensitivities are known, it may be necessary to choose an antibiotic on a 'best guess' basis, as described previously. This requires up to date information on the drug sensitivities of relevant pathogens in the locality. Familiarity with such information greatly strengthens the position of the microbiologist offering drug advice. He will also know of the prevalence of infections with various organisms, and will be in a good position to give due weight (and no more) to reports from his own laboratory.

Aim (2): To minimize the development of resistance

Drug resistance is a major consideration in antibiotic policy. Various approaches have been used, but much the most important is simply to reduce the amount or number of antibiotic(s) prescribed. The effect of antibiotic restriction may be not only to reduce the resistance of pathogens but also to reduce the prevalence of infection. Other tactics employed include the combination of drugs in the hope of delaying the emergence of resistance; the reduction of drug dosage or the time for which the drug is given; the rotation of antibiotics, and the use of many different agents. All of these ploys have their adherents: their bases are scientifically somewhat shaky, but they are all that we have to guide us at present.

If troublesome and resistant organisms become prevalent, logically devised antibiotic restriction policies may overcome the difficulty. However, the use of such solutions to solve emergent problems of antibiotic resistance is not as satisfactory as the prevention of these outbreaks. Useful contributions to the prevention of the development of resistance could be made by stopping the use of unnecessary chemotherapy, notably in unwarranted antimicrobial prophylaxis and in the use of topical chemotherapy.

Some antibiotics are more likely than others to select resistant strains of bacteria in the commensal flora of the bowel and oro-pharynx, the source of future opportunistic pathogens. An example of this phenomenon is the replacement of antibiotic-sensitive coliforms by the more antibiotic-resistant *Klebsiella* spp. or *Pseudomonas aeruginosa* as a result of ampicillin/amoxycillin or cephalosporin use. Since such organisms are particularly undesirable in areas such as intensive care units and premature baby units, a 'house rule' has been instituted at University College Hospital banning the use of these drugs in such areas. Rules, or indeed antibiotic policies as a whole, can only have local relevance and must be kept under continuing review in the light of changing circumstances.

Aim (3): Reduction of cost

Although the first requirement of chemotherapy is to select the most appropriate treatment for the individual patient, economy of expenditure is also a desirable aim, whether the patient, an insurance company or the taxpayer is paying the bill. Other considerations being equal, the cheapest drug should be preferred. As it happens, it is often true that the most clinically appropriate drug is also the cheapest, so that the first and third objectives above may be well matched.

Some figures of comparative costs of various treatments for urinary and respiratory tract infections have been given earlier in this chapter. Clearly, in the light of such figures, a policy could be devised according to locally prevailing prices which would save large sums of money without harming patients. The main savings would be made not through the very expensive but rarely prescribed drugs, but through the everyday drugs which are prescribed without much thought.

Clinicians generally need, and welcome, advice from experts on the prescription of antibiotics. In the United States of America, these experts are usually communicable diseases specialists (physicians), while in the United Kingdom, they are generally clinical microbiologists, although some interested physicians also undertake this work. The procedures followed at University College Hospital where the clinical microbiologists act as advisers on the use of antibiotics are described below.

Our aim is to achieve all three of the objectives given above: (1) optimal treatment of patients; (2) control of antibiotic resistance, and (3) low cost. We are far from complete success, but progress so far is encouraging.

We seek to provide as little laboratory encouragement to inappropriate prescribing as possible. When the clinical circumstances seem not to justify antibiotics, as, for example, in the case of intestinal pathogens from faecal samples, or the isolation of coliform organisms from varicose ulcers, antibiotic sensitivity test results are not reported. If the clinician asks why sensitivity results have not been given, we explain why we think chemotherapy inappropriate. In addition, when a report on sensitivities is appropriate, the results released to the clinician are heavily censored in the laboratory so that only a few, relatively safe, effective, environmentally 'clean', and cheap drugs are included. In the case of Group A *Streptococcus haemolyticus* or of *Streptococcus pneumoniae*, for example, we usually report only on penicillin. No more than four sensitivities are usually given for urinary pathogens. This means, for instance, that since cephalosporin sensitivities are rarely reported, this group of costly drugs is almost never used. When an organism is multiply resistant, however, full information is given.

Careful record keeping of all pathogens isolated in the laboratory and of their antibiotic sensitivities is important. We have a daily computer printout of this, and a weekly computer analysis of all significant isolates by location. This gives us early warning of apparent cross-infection, or clustering of resistant strains which may repay attention. We receive information, from the forms sent by clinicians requesting investigations, on the nature of clinical problems and on any chemotherapy being carried out. The clinicians, the medical students, or the nurses may mention problems arising on the wards.

Every day, members of the medical staff of the microbiology department do a ward round in the hospital. The first stop is at the pharmacy, to collect a list of all antibiotics which have been dispensed in the previous 24 hours. This list gives information on drug, dosage and route of administration. Anything unusual on that list occasions a visit to the patient. Any patient receiving aminoglycosides is visited in order to check that the drug is indicated and that dosage is appropriate, and to arrange for assays to be done. Dosage is then adjusted by the microbiologists. Any patient receiving cephalosporins is visited, as are all patients receiving unusual dosages or prolonged treatment with standard drugs.

Three areas are visited at least once a day: the intensive care unit, the premature baby unit and the paediatric unit. In these units, particular care is taken to prevent the use of ecologically 'dirty' drugs such as ampicillin/amoxycillin. For lack of staff, it is not yet possible for us to visit every patient receiving antibiotics, though we should like to do so. Whenever possible, we take microbiology trainees, technical staff and medical students with us on our ward rounds. Exchanges of views with the clinicians at the bedside are routine, and offer an excellent opportunity for mutual education, and for instruction of students. We also undertake some regular ward rounds with those of our clinical colleagues who face recurring problems, such as the haematologists and oncologists looking after immunologically compromised patients.

Our approach is to support our clinical colleagues and to offer constructive suggestions. Our clinical colleagues have mostly learned to trust us. If we recommend changes in treatment we do so verbally to the clinical house staff and in writing in the patient's notes, while informing the nursing staff of our intentions. We do not give instructions, only advice which the clinicians may, but usually do not, reject.

How effective is this approach? In terms of obtaining the best clinical choice of drug we are aware of many instances of having helped the clinicians to help their patients. We are now asked for advice by the clinicians very much more often than formerly, which is taken as a sign of confidence. It must be admitted, however, that some unsatisfactory antibiotic uses persist. In particular, the use of prophylactive chemotherapy in surgery is still, in my opinion, too great and somewhat irrational. In terms of protecting the environment, we have been modestly successful, mostly by preventing the use of some drugs in high dependency areas, and by achieving an overall reduction in antibiotic use. Table 3 shows that our big failure has been with amoxycillin/ampicillin, resistance to which is more common now than previously, reflecting the excessive use of these drugs. On the question of cost, we have been very pleased with our efforts. In the last three years, the cost of all drugs used at University College Hospital has more than doubled, yet the total sum spent on antimicrobial agents has not increased at all. This cannot be said of any other major group of drugs. There is still no room for complacency, however, since examination of the use of chemotherapy at this hospital suggests to me that costs could still be reduced by three-quarters without harm to patients. The saving in antibiotic costs achieved is of about the same order as the total cost of running the microbiology laboratory.

A system of the kind described here must be introduced carefully and be managed with tact and an understanding of the problems faced by clinicians. Microbiologists generally assume that receipt of a specimen is a request for a professional opinion and constitutes an invitation to visit the patient if that is thought appropriate. This may be used as a means of widening the field of interest in the wards with the consent of the clinical staff. Gradually it is seen by all to be useful for the microbiologists to have access to information from the pharmacy about the prescribing of antibiotics. A gentle introduction of such a system is likely to pay dividends.

The key to the application of any policy of this sort is the continuing education of microbiologists, laboratory technical staff, medical staff, medical students, nurses and pharmacists.

5

Infections in general practice

> She died of a fever,
>   And no-one could save her,
> And that was the end of poor Molly Malone.
>
> *Cockles and Mussels*, Traditional song, author unknown

It may reasonably be argued that many of the infections seen in general practice are similar to those found in hospitals. This is often true, but the problems of diagnosis and management differ considerably between the two situations. It is more difficult to arrange for the transport of diagnostic specimens to the laboratory from general practice than it is from the hospital. Some specialized specimens such as blood cultures or virological samples may be more difficult to collect profitably, and laboratory results are likely to be slower in their return to general practice destinations. Hospital patients are often more unwell than their counterparts being managed at home. This is partly because patients who are more ill are sent to hospital for that reason; partly because hospital patients as a group are older, more frail and more likely to have other complicating diseases such as diabetes, and partly because of the impact of diagnostic or therapeutic procedures carried out in hospitals (e.g. intravenous infusions, immunosuppression, steroid treatment, and surgical wounds). Additionally, the infecting organisms in hospitals may be of unusual or more virulent types, or be more antibiotic resistant than those in domiciliary practice.

85

Thus, although there is much in common between infections occur-ring in patients at home and those occurring in patients in hospital, it will, to some extent, be proper for them to be investigated and man-aged differently. Accordingly, in this chapter I will discuss infections occurring in patients at home, and in the next, the different problems arising in hospital infections.

Use of the microbiology laboratory

All medical students are taught not to begin treatment until a diagnosis has been made, and that antibiotic choice should be governed by the antibiotic sensitivities of the pathogen. In general practice, the indications for sending specimens to the microbiology laboratory may be different from those taught in hospital. Specimens may well be sent for reasons of self-education of general practitioners, for the instruc-tion of trainees, for reassurance of the patient or his relatives, for epi-demiological interest, or in pursuit of some research objective. Aside from these perfectly legitimate reasons, the question of when a general practitioner should use the microbiology laboratory is discussed below. Throat swabs should be collected and sent (in transport medium to prevent drying) to the laboratory from any case of pharyngitis which may require antibiotic treatment. Only those yielding haemoly-tic streptococci of Lancefield's Group A or *Corynebacterium diph-theriae* may need antimicrobial chemotherapy (see section on respirat-ory tract infection, below). Nose swabs very rarely yield useful information in general practice. Ear swabs (in transport medium) have some limited value in the management of patients with acute otitis media, but only if the ear drum is perforated. The management of otitis externa will seldom be affected by laboratory findings.

Sputum samples and specimens of presumed paranasal sinus con-tents are of diagnostic value only if collected freshly and delivered to the laboratory very quickly. They are of no value if not frankly purul-ent on inspection or if collected from patients receiving antibiotics. Even in hospital, sputum bacteriology is often very unrewarding. In my own laboratory, we do not accept sputum samples from out-patients or from general practice because of the very poor yield of use-ful information for effort expended, and because of the danger, greater in this than in any other investigation, of reporting misleading results.

An exception is the culture of sputum for tubercle bacilli but this must be specifically requested.

Diagnostic urine samples should always be sent from patients with frequency and dysuria. Only about half of such patients will be found to have significant bacteriuria which alone may justify the use of antimicrobial chemotherapy. Treatment need not await the results of sensitivity testing because resistance to antibiotics is relatively uncommon among urinary pathogens in general practice (Table 3). If the pathogen is resistant to the drug being given, the treatment can be changed later, and, when no pathogen is isolated from further samples, it can safely be stopped. Urine samples should be sent one week and five weeks after treatment to check for clearance of the infection. Failure of appropriate chemotherapy for UTI, repeated episodes of bacteriologically proved UTI in an adult, or a single episode of proved UTI in a child are indications for referral to a specialist.

Stool specimens (rather than rectal swabs if faeces can be obtained) may be sent to the laboratory to establish the diagnosis in patients with diarrhoea, or for epidemiological reasons, but not to guide antibiotic treatment which is only very rarely justified.

Wound swabs (in transport medium) should be sent for culture only if the result is likely to modify treatment. Swabs from the intact skin overlying a closed abscess are unlikely to give useful information. Once an abscess is draining freely, there is unlikely to be an indication for the use of antibiotics and so culture of the pus will yield little useful information in general practice. (The more spectacular abscesses are likely to be managed in hospitals.)

Ulcerated lesions should be cultured bacteriologically only if there is clinical evidence of inflammation (pain, swelling, redness, local warmth, loss of function) otherwise, harmless commensal organisms may be treated as pathogens. This means that there is little to be gained from sampling most varicose ulcers or bed sores, but that useful information may be gained from sampling impetigo for bacteriological culture, or suspected herpes simplex infections and shingles for virological examination (special methods apply, see Chapter 3).

The investigation of unexplained fever is always potentially difficult. As has already been discussed (in Chapter 2) it should be carefully planned and not be undertaken in a piecemeal fashion. If the first few, relatively simple investigations have not established the diagnosis, the patient should be referred urgently for hospital assessment.

Far more infections are caused by viruses in general practice than is the case in hospital practice. Many of the viral infections of the respiratory and gastro-intestinal tracts are self-limiting and relatively minor. If the general practitioner has the interest to investigate such episodes, it is important to begin the process very early in the illness (Chapter 3) and to see that specimens for virological culture are accompanied by the first 'acute' specimen of clotted blood for antibody studies, with a second 'convalescent' blood sample to follow 10 to 14 days later. Without such antibody studies, it will not often be possible to establish whether a virus cultured from the patient is related to the illness. Serological tests, whether virological or not, very often require two samples for comparison, one collected early in the course of the disease and the second, one to two weeks later. This is because a single antibody level is usually not interpretable, but changes in antibody level may be related to the course of clinical events. A few serological tests however, such as those for syphilis and for glandular fever (infectious mononucleosis) may require only a single sample.

Respiratory tract infection

The majority of acute respiratory tract infections seen in general practice are caused by viruses, bacteria being involved as secondary invaders in many instances. Most of these episodes are self-limiting and do not pose a serious threat to the patient.

Acute pharyngitis is nearly always viral and requires symptomatic treatment only. Pharyngitis or tonsillitis may be associated with the presence of *Streptococcus haemolyticus* (Group A) either causally or coincidentally. Some such patients may benefit from the use of penicillin (to which the organism is always sensitive) or erythromycin. Antibiotics should not be given to patients with pharyngitis unless *S. haemolyticus* (Group A) is present: nor should they be given if symptoms are mild. Except in outbreaks, it is a mistake, in my opinion, to treat the 5—15% of the population who may be carrying this organism just because of the possibility that it may be a strain capable of causing glomerulonephritis, rheumatic fever or scarlet fever. When treatment is to be given, it must be with adequate chemotherapy. Penicillin V should be given to adults, in appropriate cases, in a dosage of 500 mg,

6-hourly, by mouth, for at least seven days. Drugs which are of uncertain effectiveness, such as the tetracyclines, should not be used. Ampicillin/amoxycillin is less effective than penicillin V and is very likely to cause side effects if the pharyngitis is due to glandular fever. In prosperous societies, diphtheria is now a rarity, but it should not be forgotten. It may present with pharyngitis as part of the clinical picture. It will not be possible to culture the organism from a swab taken after antibiotic treatment has started.

Sinusitis is a clinical and radiological diagnosis. The problem is largely one of restoring free drainage by appropriate means, rather than of chemotherapy. If antimicrobial treatment is needed, amoxycillin, co-trimoxazole or a tetracycline are likely to be effective. In otitis media, amoxycillin or co-trimoxazole will be appropriate. In this condition, the objectives of treatment are pain relief and the prevention of rupture of the ear drum. Otitis externa is unlikely to be helped by antibiotics except perhaps in acute episodes. The mixed microbial flora isolated from the auditory meatus are commonly colonizing, not invading, the moist skin. Painful meatal boils may require chemotherapy.

Coughing is a common symptom, present in many conditions. It is not, of itself, a justification for drug treatment, still less for the use of antibiotics. Most episodes of acute cough are associated with minor viral infections of the larynx and trachea and require no antimicrobial treatment. Some are associated with more widespread infections such as acute bronchitis. In these conditions, there is little evidence of benefit from the use of antibiotics in terms of symptomatic improvement, improvement in physical signs and respiratory function, or prevention of the relatively infrequent complications (Howie and Hutchison, 1978). If antibiotics must be used, amoxycillin, oxytetracycline or co-trimoxazole is a good choice.

In general practice, 'primary atypical pneumonia' caused by *Mycoplasma pneumoniae* is quite common. The diagnosis is a clinical one which may be supported by culture of the pathogen from the sputum (rarely performed), by serological evidence of antibody response to the mycoplasma, or possibly, by the presence of circulating cold agglutinins. Treatment should involve either erythromycin or a tetracycline.

Chronic bronchitis should not be regarded as a simple infection although it clearly has an infective component, if only at times when an acute episode is superimposed on the longstanding process. Many of these acute episodes are initiated by viral infections, but go on to secondary bacterial infection for which antibiotic treatment may be appropriate in an attempt to reduce the amount or purulence of sputum and so avoid additional respiratory function deterioration. Co-trimoxazole, oxytetracycline or amoxycillin may be used.

Bronchopneumonia is quite a common condition, usually following viral infection in small children or old people, and often being associated in the old with taking to bed because of some other illness. Mobilization and expectoration of the purulent sputum accumulating at the lung bases, either by the patient's own efforts or with the assistance of physiotherapy, are important: antibiotics probably less so. Nonetheless, antibiotics will rarely be withheld from such patients. Chloramphenicol, amoxycillin, co-trimoxazole or oxytetracycline may be used. Poor respiratory function, carbon dioxide retention or failure to respond to treatment are indications for hospitalization.

Lobar pneumonia is much less common than bronchopneumonia. It is generally caused by the pneumococcus (*Streptococcus pneumoniae*) and should be treated with penicillin G, parenterally. This means that patients with lobar pneumonia should usually be treated in hospital.

Children with acute respiratory tract infections may, on occasion, be suffering from measles, respiratory syncytial virus infection, whooping cough or *Haemophilus influenzae* infection of the epiglottis. Measles may be complicated by otitis media, bronchitis or bronchopneumonia. These complications should be watched for and treated on their merits, but prophylactic antibiotics should not be given. Infections with respiratory syncytial virus (RSV) tend to affect babies. They occur mostly in winter and in large outbreaks. They may give rise (rarely) to sudden respiratory obstruction, some fatal cases of which are reported as 'cot deaths'. Antibiotics will not help in RSV infection. Suspected cases should be sent to the accident and emergency department of a hospital to be assessed by a paediatrician. Rapid virological diagnosis is available for this condition. Whooping cough is a very trying condition for the patient and for the parents. Some cases are caused by viruses, and some by *Bordetella pertussis* which can be isolated by the culture of pernasal swabs or of cough plates early in the episode. Antibiotics (chloramphenicol, amoxycillin or erythromycin) probably affect the course of the infection only in the first few days. Many cases are brought for advice only after some days, by which time it is unlikely that antibiotics will help. *Haemophilus influenzae* epiglottitis is a rare condition, the importance of which is due to its propensity to cause sudden respiratory obstruction. It will respond to chloramphenicol or, sometimes, to amoxycillin. Children in whom this, or any other, cause of croup is suspected should be sent to the accident and emergency department of a nearby hospital, at once.

Gastro-intestinal infections

These are very common in general practice. Very frequently, no diagnosis is made, even when appropriate investigations are made. Some of the episodes are probably intoxications ('food poisoning') rather than infections, although the irritant may well be elaborated by a micro-organism. Examples of this include the potent exotoxin produced by some strains of *Staphylococcus aureus* in contaminated food and the toxins produced by *Clostridium perfringens (welchii)* and *Bacillus cereus*. Apart from these, some enteroviruses; some rotaviruses; *Campylobacter jejuni*; some serotypes of *Escherichia coli*; *Salmonella* spp.; *Shigella* spp.; *Vibrio parahaemolyticus*; *Vibrio cholerae*, and *Giardia lamblia* and other intestinal parasites may all be involved, although with different degrees of likelihood in different parts of the world.

The identification of these micro-organisms in foodstuffs, water or the dejecta of patients suffering from diarrhoea or vomiting is important on public health grounds. Most countries have, or are setting up, public health laboratory services linked to diagnostic laboratories to faciltate the tracing of outbreaks of such infections and to disseminate relevant information to doctors, veterinary workers and those working in agriculture, catering and the food preparation industries. General practitioners should notify the public health authorities of cases of suspected food poisoning and should send relevant material, including remains of food, to the laboratory. The laboratory may be able to make a bacteriological or virological diagnosis and this will help the doctor to set his patient's mind at rest regarding the cause of his symptoms, to advise about the desirability of clearance checks in food handlers before returning to work and even, in rare cases, to decide upon the desirability of isolation of the patient. It will help only rarely in guiding the choice of antimicrobial chemotherapy.

The management of diarrhoea and vomiting should be concerned with control of symptoms, maintenance of hydration and of acid—base balance and replacement of depleted minerals. Severe cases should be managed in hospital because of need for constant observation and biochemical analyses. In most of the infections listed above, antibiotics have no application or only a very limited role. *Salmonella* infections should be treated with antibiotics only if the organism gives rise to a septicaemia, because their use otherwise does not shorten the symptomatic period or reduce the period of faecal excretion of the organism. For similar reasons, bacillary dysentery (caused by *Shigella* spp.) should be treated with antibiotics only in the rare instances of systemic spread of the organism, or if the organism is one of the infrequent strains of *Shigella dysenteriae* which produces a potent neurotoxin. Amoebic dysentery (caused by *Entamoeba histolytica*) and giardiasis should be treated with appropriate chemotherapy. Infections with *Vibrio parahaemolyticus* are usually derived from shellfish and are self-limiting and of short duration, although unpleasant. Antibiotics do not help in this case. Even in cholera, the main problems are of hydration and mineral balance. The clinical course of the disease and the period of carriage of the causative *Vibrio cholerae* are shortened by only a few hours by treatment with the drugs usually used, tetracycline or co-trimoxazole. Cholera and enteric fever are usually managed in hospital.

Enteric fever (caused by *Salmonella typhi*, *S. paratyphi*, A, B or C and, occasionally, by other species of *Salmonella*) is really a septicaemia rather than an intestinal infection, although the portal of entry is through the Peyer's patches in the small intestine, and diarrhoea is only featured very briefly, if at all. Patients with enteric fever should be treated with antibiotics. The established drugs are chloramphenicol and co-trimoxazole. More recently, claims have been made for the usefulness of amoxycillin and mecillinam. Antibiotics are used to produce a cure, to reduce the length and severity of the disease, and in the hope of reducing the likelihood of patients becoming longterm carriers of *S. typhi* or other enteric pathogens.

Urinary tract infection

Most urinary tract infection (UTI) is asymptomatic, and only about half of patients complaining of dysuria and frequency prove to have UTI. This means that all practitioners should have this diagnostic possibility in mind and should send urine samples to the laboratory, seeking the demonstration of 'significant bacteriuria' (more than 100 000 of one type of organism per millilitre in two samples of urine) which alone establishes the diagnosis of UTI.

Symptomatic patients with UTI should be treated with a short course of appropriate chemotherapy. In general practice UTI, the cure rate with any of the usual drugs is so high (80—85%) that it is almost impossible to demonstrate the superiority of one to another. The choice can therefore be made on other grounds: oral administration, acceptability to the patient, low incidence of side effects, mildness of side effects, low level of resistance among urinary pathogens (Table 3) and cost. In my opinion, a sulphonamide or co-trimoxazole is likely to give the most satisfactory results. Treatment failures, or patients with recurrent UTI, should be referred for specialist assessment.

Children with UTI present several problems. They may have apparently unrelated symptoms (e.g. crying bouts, fits, unexplained fever, vomiting, resumed bedwetting, failure to thrive) or they may not be symptomatic at all. Any child under the age of five years brought to see a general practitioner should therefore have a urine sample cultured. Very young children may pose problems in specimen collection. Many treated episodes of UTI in children recur (70% reinfected within two years) so that longterm follow-up is needed. Most importantly, anything interfering with the normal growth and development of the kidneys of prepubertal children (such as acute pyelonephritis progressing to chronic pyelonephritis) may give rise to progressive renal function deficit or even, in severe cases, to chronic renal failure. Any episode of UTI in a child up to the age of puberty (say, thirteen years), whether symptomatic or not, should be treated and cleared. All children with one documented attack of UTI should be referred for urological assessment and follow-up for at least two years, in such a way that reinfections can be detected and treated. Children who are shown to have vesico-ureteric reflux and who have had even one episode of UTI, will benefit from longterm, low dosage, antibiotic prophylaxis with co-trimoxazole or nitrofurantoin (Smellie *et al.*, 1978).

All pregnant women should have a urine sample examined for significant bacteriuria at their first attendance in pregnancy, because those with untreated UTI have a high probability of developing acute pyelonephritis later in pregnancy or in the puerperium, and because babies born to bacteriuric mothers have a lower birth weight than those born to the uninfected. In pregnancy, cure rates of UTI treated with short courses of antibiotics are about 75% compared with the 80—85% expected in non-pregnant women. In the first six months of pregnancy, sulphonamide or amoxycillin may be used with good effect. Sulphonamide (and co-trimoxazole) should not be used in the last weeks of pregnancy for fear of precipitating hyperbilirubinaemia or even kernicterus in the neonate. Pregnant women who fail a single, short course of appropriate treatment for UTI should be investigated urologically six months after delivery (Leigh *et al.*, 1968).

There is no objective evidence that UTI occurring in non-pregnant adults does any harm other than perhaps causing troublesome symptoms. It is, therefore, uncertain whether men or non-pregnant women discovered to have asymptomatic UTI should be treated. Personally, I recommend treatment of such patients, partly because I have a feeling that the urinary tract should properly be sterile, and partly because I am not satisfied that just because UTI has not been shown to be harmful, it can be regarded as harmless. I make an exception in the case of patients with indwelling catheters and UTI in which experience has shown me that antibiotic treatment will either fail, or succeed only for the original pathogen to be replaced by another. I also leave untreated asymptomatic patients found to have UTI caused by very low grade pathogens such as *Pseudomonas aeruginosa*, since such patients, in my experience, nearly always prove to have structural and functional abnormalities of the urinary tract such that treatment, even if successful, results in the replacement of the initial, relatively kindly organism by another, often more virulent, pathogen.

Genito-urinary infections

The venereal diseases syphilis, gonorrhoea and non-gonococcal urethritis quite often present to the general practitioner, and even more often figure in the differential diagnosis of problems seen by him. This group of infections may present considerable diagnostic, therapeutic and epidemiological problems, not to mention medico-legal difficulties. For these reasons, I suggest that patients suspected of suffering from any of these infections should be referred to a venereologist for assessment. No attempt should be made to 'treat' such patients with antibiotics without a firm diagnosis having been established. Mixed infections are common. The treatment of these conditions has been well reviewed by Ridgway (1980).

Vaginal candidiasis may be caused by any member of the *Candida* genus of yeasts, not only by the commonest, *Candida albicans*. These yeasts can be isolated from the genital tract of far more women than suffer from the vaginal symptoms often attributed to them. Unless a woman from whom the organism is isolated is suffering from vulvovaginitis, she should not be treated. Infected patients' vaginal swabs will yield a heavy growth of yeasts rather than a scanty growth, and a Gram-stained smear of vaginal mucosa will show the fungus in its invasive hyphal form as well as in the yeast form. High vaginal swabs collected in order to establish this or other microbiological diagnoses, should be sent to the laboratory in transport medium. This will ensure that any *Trichomonas vaginalis* present remain in a motile state so that they can be seen in a wet preparation under the microscope. The sexual partners of patients found to have trichomoniasis or candidiasis should also be examined and, perhaps, be treated in order to prevent recurrence due to the organism being passed to and fro ('ping-pong' infection).

Request forms accompanying vaginal swabs to the laboratory should indicate the nature of the clinical problem (e.g. vaginal discharge, pelvic pain), and also the precise site sampled (e.g. high vaginal swab, cervical swab). This is necessary in order to help the laboratory to provide useful information. Swabs collected from patients with vaginitis or vaginal discharge are examined for *Trichomonas vaginalis* and *Candida* spp., whereas those collected from patients in the puerperium or following gynaecological surgery will be examined for quite different organisms using other techniques. High vaginal swabs are often inadequate for the diagnosis of gonorrhoea, for which cervical, urethral and rectal swabs are needed, these being cultured differently. Inadequate specimens or insufficient information will result in the laboratory failing to provide as much diagnostic support as is possible.

Puerperal or postoperative endometritis is a quite different problem. It is likely to be caused by *Streptococcus haemolyticus* (Group A), *Clostridium perfringens (welchii)*, anaerobic streptococci or other anaerobes. The laboratory should be told the nature of the problem so that appropriate cultures can be set up. Similarly, if enough relevant information is provided, the laboratory can investigate for *Mycoplasma hominis* or *Ureaplasma urealyticum* if this is not part of local laboratory routine. Knowledge that a patient with cervical discharge has an intra-uterine contraceptive device in position will cause the laboratory to look for unusual organisms, such as *Actinomyces israeli*, sometimes isolated from such patients.

Virological samples should be collected from patients suspected of suffering from genital herpes infection. This diagnosis can be confirmed by a virus laboratory within hours if an electron microscope is available, or in two to three days by tissue culture. Patients found to have genital herpes should be referred either to a gynaecologist or to a venereologist.

Other infections

Skin lesions should be examined microbiologically only if they show signs of infection. If this rule is adhered to, the results coming back to the practitioner may have some clinical relevance and be a reasonable basis for guiding antibiotic choice. If treatment is decided upon, antibiotics should be given systemically rather than topically. This will ensure penetration of antibiotic to the site of the infection (which is often not as superficial as it appears), will reduce the likelihood of local antibiotic hypersensitivity reactions, and will minimize the emergence of antibiotic-resistant bacteria which otherwise may occur through exposure to subinhibitory concentrations of a locally applied drug. The use of ointments containing steroids plus antibiotics is, in my opinion, to be deplored: if antibiotics are needed they should be given systemically, and if they are not needed they should not be given.

Moist, weeping lesions such as varicose ulcers, nappy rash and umbilical erosions are virtually always colonized by Gram-negative bacteria and sometimes by yeasts. They should not be cultured or treated with antibiotics unless they are clinically infected. If the lesion can be kept dry by the use of appropriate dressings, exposure to the air or the use of absorbent talcum powder (perhaps containing antiseptics), the colonization by the usual organisms will cease and the lesion will have a chance to heal. Similarly, moist wounds such as discharging sinuses are almost invariably colonized by Gram-negative bacilli. The inner dressing, rather than a swab, should be sent for culture if there is any question of anaerobic infection, actinomycosis or tuberculosis. If wound toilet with antiseptics such as hypochlorite solutions is appropriate, the wound should subsequently be dried and covered with a dry dressing.

The use of antibiotics in relation to wounds should be directed at prevention of spread of infection through the tissues, and at prevention of bloodstream spread in closed infections. The use of antibiotics to try to sterilize a closed abscess should be discouraged as it is most unlikely to be effective. Once an abscess has been drained, either by rupture or by incision, there is no further use for antibiotics because local or distant spread is no longer likely.

Meningitis will nowadays always be treated in hospital. Very commonly, however, patients seen in hospital with meningitis have received antibiotics at home before it became apparent what was amiss. This has caused a whole generation of medical teachers to complain to medical students about the irresponsible use of antibiotics by general practitioners obscuring the diagnosis when the patient is finally admitted to hospital. This purist line about the inadvisability of using antibiotics until a diagnosis has been made is not to be dismissed, but there is no gainsaying the obvious benefit which many patients with bacterial meningitis have received from 'misdirected and suboptimal' chemotherapy.

6

Infections in hospitals

Every physician almost hath his favourite disease.

Tom Jones, book 2, chapter 9, Henry Fielding (1707—1754)

As was noted at the beginning of the previous chapter, there is much in common between infections occurring inside hospitals and outside them. Nonetheless, there are problems which are worse in hospitals than elsewhere, and there are problems which are virtually confined to hospital practice. The problems of degree are concerned with the susceptibility of hospital patients to infection because of old age and frailty and because of the likelihood that they will be suffering from other conditions which will make them both more infection prone and more difficult to treat when infected. There is also the probability that hospital patients will include those most seriously infected, either because they were sent to hospital for that very reason, or because of the increased chance of infection associated with diagnostic and therapeutic procedures such as surgical operations, catheterization, immunosuppression, transfusion, irradiation and the effect of drugs. There is also an accumulation in hospitals of a bacterial flora containing more virulent organisms, organisms with a greater than usual capacity to spread from person to person, and organisms with more antibiotic resistance than those outside. The main problem, almost confined to hospital practice, is that of cross-infection.

There is no unique difference between the bacterial flora of lesions occurring in hospital and those occurring outside. The point may be exemplified by consideration of urinary tract infection (UTI) diagnosed in hospital. The source of the pathogens causing UTI is the patient's own faecal flora. A patient whose UTI is first diagnosed in hospital may have been infected (from his own faecal flora) before he was admitted to hospital. Alternatively, he may have acquired his UTI in hospital shortly after admission, the pathogen being derived from his own (still predominantly domiciliary) faecal flora. A little later on, his faecal flora will have been replaced by organisms more characteristic of the hospital environment, and this may have given rise to UTI caused by an endogenous organism of a 'hospital' type. If he was subjected to catheterization or operation, the possibility of exogenous UTI arises, such infections being caused either by the environmental flora or by 'cross-infection' from other patients in the clinical unit. The nature and degree of antibiotic resistance of such environmental and cross-infecting strains will vary from unit to unit and from time to time, and will reflect local clinical practices and antibiotic usage. When, in due course, our patient, with or without UTI, was discharged from hospital, he would take his 'hospital' urinary bacterial flora with him, so potentially changing the local domiciliary bacterial flora. In other words, there is a constant exchange of organisms, both commensals and pathogens, between hospitals and the communities which they serve. Clinical decisions taken in one environment affect the ecological situation locally and at a distance. From the point of view of the patient with UTI, it does not make any difference where his urinary pathogen came from, his infection should be treated on its merits. Nonetheless, the nature and antibiotic resistance of the pathogen will depend on its derivation, and so this will affect the choice of treatment.

Infecting organisms

Studies of hospital infection have tended, until very recently, to concentrate on infected surgical wounds. This is a relatively new problem, because surgery was a rare undertaking, except for the treatment of battle injuries, until modern times, when the development of anaesthetics, of adequate treatment for shock, and of blood transfusion, transformed the scene. Many of the major advances in our knowledge of surgical sepsis and its prevention have been derived from studies undertaken to minimize postoperative infection in surgically treated war wounds. As time went by, antiseptic surgery (introduced by Lord Lister, an ex-member of the staff at University College Hospital) reduced the frequency of wound infections, and this was reduced further by aseptic technique. The surgical infection rate was still appreciable and the increasing skills of bacteriologists led to the realization of the importance of cross-infection with haemolytic streptococci or, more recently, with *Staphylococcus aureus*. Much more stringent operating theatre disciplines and surgical wound dressing routines, introduced during and after the Second World War, gradually reduced the significance of staphylococcal cross-infection. This trend was reinforced by the ability of the pharmaceutical industry, from 1960 onwards, to produce potent new antibiotics capable of treating staphylococcal sepsis. Clinicians became overconfident because the problems of wound infection and of staphylococcal cross-infection had been largely (although not completely) overcome.

It was not until midway through the nineteen sixties, that clinicians and microbiologists began to realize that a new, much less tractable, problem had arisen. Hospital infections were now much more commonly caused by Gram-negative bacilli than formerly. Organisms such as the coliform bacilli, *Proteus* spp. and *Pseudomonas aeruginosa* were becoming important hospital pathogens. This happened partly because of more radical and ambitious surgical procedures; partly because of the use of catheters and intravenous infusions; partly because of the use of drugs such as corticosteroids and immunosuppressive agents; partly because of the control of the more pathogenic Gram-positive bacteria, and partly because of the increasing use of antibiotics which created an ecological vacuum into which the Gram-negative bacilli could move. New bacteriological studies were undertaken, new clinical and nursing procedures adopted, and new antibiotics active against Gram-negative bacteria were introduced, with the result that by the mid-nineteen seventies, the problem of Gram-negative infections in hospitals began to recede. Such infections remain common in our hospitals, however, and the problems of their management are compounded by increasing antibiotic resistance among hospital strains of Gram-negative pathogens.

A new problem began to be more widely recognized in the nineteen seventies: the pathogenic potential of the anaerobic organisms of the human bowel. It gradually became apparent that coliform organisms and faecal anaerobes were causing infections. Where only one of these types of organism was involved, the infections were quite easy to manage, but it was found that mixed aerobic and anaerobic infections of abdominal surgical wounds or of gynaecological surgical wounds presented major difficulties. This realization depended upon much improved technical methods of isolating and identifying anaerobic bacteria from clinical material. (In places where laboratory facilities for isolation of anaerobic organisms are not available, the use of the human nose is a great help: if a lesion smells foul it is infected with anaerobes.) Increased awareness of the importance of coliform and anaerobe sepsis has led to the devising of various regimes of prophylactic antimicrobial therapy by the instillation of drugs into the wound and by their administration parenterally. I dislike this development because of the large increase in antibiotic use entailed, and the subsequent likelihood of adding to the pressure of selection of antibiotic-resistant organisms. None of the antibiotic prophylactic regimes have been shown to be markedly better than the instillation of povidone iodine into the wound at operation: a safe, effective and cheap measure which does not jeopardize the use of the antibiotics (Stokes *et al.*, 1977). When antibiotics are used prophylactically, they should be given at operation and for not more than 24 hours thereafter.

With increasing use of central venous catheterization ('long lines') and of peritoneal dialysis, which are often combined with the use of broad spectrum antibiotics, infections with opportunistic fungi, particularly *Candida* spp., are becoming more common in hospitals.

Source, transmission and portal of entry of organisms

In considering any infection with a view to its prevention, it is sensible to consider the source of the causative organisms, the means of transmission to the patient, and the portal of entry. Nearly all organisms causing infection in hospitals are derived from human beings. The most important source is the patient's own flora, whether derived from mouth, intestine or skin. Less frequently, organisms are derived either from lesions or from the commensal flora of other patients, of nursing or medical staff, or of visitors. Infecting organisms may derive from animal sources, as sometimes happens with intestinal infections. There is almost no organism colonizing man which seems incapable of causing hospital infection.

The route of transmission of hospital infections varies from infection to infection. It may be through the air, as commonly happens with respiratory tract infections when coughing or sneezing by patients, staff, or others may lead to droplets carrying microbes being shed into the atmosphere. Some of these droplets dry out leaving organisms in much smaller droplet nuclei or floating free. Some settle in the dust on the floor where they may be joined by organisms on shed hairs or skin flakes. The dust on the floor will be disturbed by people's feet, bed-making, ward cleaning and so on, leaving many of the organisms resuspended in the air, free to blow towards the patient. A second means of transmission of infection is by personal contact, whether between patients or between patient and nurse, doctor, other staff or visitors. The closer the personal contact, the readier the transmission of pathogens. Ingestion of infected food or drink offers a third route for transfer of pathogens. Another means of micro-organism transfer of great potential importance, is by the agency of contaminated objects (fomites) such as surgical instruments, hypodermic syringes or needles, dressings, intravenous fluids, crockery and cutlery, bedding or baths. Transfer by insect or other animal bite should be rare in well conducted hospitals.

The portal of entry of infection varies from one type of infection to another, and will be partly determined by the route of transmission. Airborne infection will mostly enter the patient by inhalation and will, therefore, mostly affect the respiratory tract. Organisms carried in the air may also contaminate wounds either in the operating theatre or in the ward. Personal contact may transfer organisms causing skin infections, infections of burns or wounds, and even sexually transmitted diseases (although not often in hospitals, it is to be hoped). Infected food or drink will cause intestinal infections. Infections transferred by inanimate objects may be enormously varied, including skin conditions derived from baths, intestinal infections from crockery and cutlery, hepatitis from syringes and needles, septicaemia from intravenous fluids, and wound sepsis from surgical instruments or dressings. Insect or other animal bites will cause local and perhaps systemic infections, depending on the nature of the pathogen transmitted.

Outbreaks of infection

Considerations such as those outlined above indicate the lines to be followed when a number of cases of infection occur at the same time. The person investigating such a situation will first review the reported cases, and will then seek out any others not yet reported. It will then be necessary to consider whether they really are cases of infection (often this is not so) and, if they are, to try to determine their nature by asking questions such as those listed below.

(1)   Are the infecting organisms all apparently the same, or are they different? If they are all the same, there is *prima facie* evidence of cross-infection, but if they are different, there is not.

(2)   What was the sequence of cases?

(3)   Were they all operated upon in one operating session?

(4)   Are the patients all in the care of one team?

(5)   Were they all having their wounds dressed by one nurse?

(6)   Was there a breakdown of sterilization processes at the relevant time which would have affected the production of sterile instruments, catheters, dressings or intravenous fluids?

Detective investigations of this sort have a certain theoretical attraction, but, in my experience, often prove disappointing. There is often very little evidence that so-called infected patients really are infected. When they are infected, it is usually with several unrelated organisms and there is no evidence of cross-infection. The search then becomes one for lapses in measures designed to minimize infection. This usually leads to the discovery of several different shortcomings in medical and nursing procedures, any one of which may have had something to do with causing infection. Despite these disappointments, however, microbiologists should always respond quickly and energetically to news of possible outbreaks of infection. After all, the next one may be genuine, and it is important to get on top of real outbreaks quickly, and to maintain the enthusiasm of nurses and doctors for preventive measures.

Mention was made in Chapter 2 of laboratory techniques for identifying different strains of common pathogens by bacteriophage typing, bacteriocine production and serotyping. Such differentiation of strains from apparent outbreaks may be of the utmost importance in investigating what may prove to be cross-infection. Laboratory staff should be watching for clusters of cases in one location, or possible outbreaks among the patients of one team of clinicians. In large laboratories, computers help to keep track of infections and to give early warning of indications of impending outbreaks. The laboratory fills an important rôle in investigations of suspected outbreaks by isolating and 'fingerprinting' pathogens from patients, staff and the environment. The microbiologist should therefore take charge of the investigation from the start and should be notified before (not after) specimens are taken, so that he can ensure that they are appropriate. Clinicians should not begin the investigations themselves because they lack the specialized knowledge and experience required. Again, my experience has been that the microbiologists have more often told the clinicians that an outbreak was in full swing than the other way around.

The key to these epidemiological problems of hospital infection is to emphasize the importance of prevention. There should be a Control of Infection Committee, one major activity of which should be the production and updating of an Infection Control Manual appropriate to local circumstances. This manual would lay down the infection prevention procedures to be used in the hospital, and these should be adhered to by all staff. The subject of infection prevention in hospitals will be dealt with more fully in Chapter 8.

Use of the laboratory

Diagnostic laboratories will usually be used much more heavily by hospital doctors than by those engaged in primary care because of the greater complexity of the clinical problems dealt with by the former. Specimens will be sent as part of a screening process for otherwise undetectable infection, as part of the diagnostic process, and to monitor the patient's response to treatment.

Screening for unsuspected infection can easily get out of hand and should be discussed with the laboratory staff. It should be done when the number of cases discovered will be appreciable, when neglect of the infection will be harmful to the patient or to others, and when treatment may do some good. Procedures which will yield very few positive diagnoses should be eschewed. Examples of such procedures in Britain would be the routine chest X-ray of all hospital inpatients in the search for pulmonary tuberculosis, and the routine performance of syphilis serology on all patients. In each of these cases, the yield of positives would be very small. Screening of selected groups of patients, for example chest X-ray for tuberculosis of immigrants from areas in which the disease is more prevalent, the testing of blood donors for freedom from syphilis or hepatitis B, or the testing of pregnant women for significant bacteriuria, may be more productive. It will usually be sensible to agree policy for particular units with the laboratory staff. At University College Hospital for example, we have an agreed policy whereby every infant admitted to the neonatal intensive care unit has swabs of throat, ear, umbilicus and rectum screened for haemolytic streptococci and *Pseudomonas aeruginosa* in order to control the spread of these organisms among the patients and staff and to give early warning of any lapse in aseptic technique. These cultures are repeated every week on every baby in the unit. This policy has been agreed because it has been found to be of value. It is, however, expensive to run (approximately £20 000 per year) and involves a substantial amount of work for nurses and for the laboratory. Adoption of similar schemes elsewhere in the hospital without evidence of benefit would inundate the laboratory with useless work and cost a great deal of money.

The diagnostic work of the laboratory is more difficult to evaluate, if only because of its variety. It has been suggested that certain types of specimen yield very little useful information (examples being non-purulent sputum or sputum samples from patients receiving antibiotics, nose swabs other than for epidemiological studies, swabs from the throat of patients with unexplained fever and cultures of uninfected varicose ulcers). It has also been suggested that the despatch of specimens to the laboratory with insufficient clinical information is a waste of effort all round. As indicated in Chapter 2, the laboratory investigation of clinical problems should be carefully planned. Whenever possible the plan of investigations of standard clinical situations should be agreed between the clinicians and the laboratory staff, with the aim of maximizing the useful diagnostic information, minimizing unproductive laboratory work and obtaining value for money. In this way, to the advantage of all concerned, the microbiologists in my hospital have agreed the investigative protocols for patients with suspected sexually transmitted diseases with colleagues in the Department of Genito-urinary Medicine, and the investigative procedures for ailing babies with colleagues in Neonatal Medicine.

Whenever possible, treatment should be withheld until laboratory results are available, or at any rate until diagnostic samples have been collected. Failure to do this may result in worse harm to patients than would follow from waiting. Junior clinical staff are often in more of a hurry to initiate treatment than is clinically indicated. This is partly due to inexperience, partly due to misconceptions about the dreadful outcome of untreated infections and partly due to romantic ideas about the instantaneous lifesaving efficacy of antibiotics. It is the responsibility of senior clinical staff and of clinical microbiologists to restore a sense of proportion and to restrain the therapeutic enthusiasm of the less experienced.

The work of the microbiology laboratory in monitoring treatment outcome is of two kinds: (1) checking that the pathogen has been eliminated and keeping a watch for relapse or reinfection, and (2) assaying antibiotic levels to ensure that sufficient drug is given and that toxic accumulation of antibiotic does not occur. In this context, clinical microbiologists may be able to advise on dosage of antibiotics and on when to stop treatment.

Septicaemia

Patients in hospital often have organisms circulating in the bloodstream. This may be a harmless bacteraemia associated with some localized sepsis, the bacteria 'spilling over' into the bloodstream, and may be of diagnostic value under circumstances in which it is not possible to isolate the pathogen from the original lesion. Bacteraemia of this type usually subsides as treatment of the source of the bacteria takes effect. Although there may be a higher mortality associated with infections giving rise to bacteraemia, this is not caused by the presence of the bacteria in the blood, but by the fact that 'overspill' of bacteria is associated with the more severe infections. Treatment should be directed to the original locus of infection and need not be modified because of the presence of bacteraemia.

In septicaemia, the bacterial load in the bloodstream is heavier and the micro-organisms may actually be multiplying as they spread. Metastatic abscess formation is common. Appropriate treatment for the originating locus of infection plus vigorous treatment for the septicaemia should be given. This treatment should be commenced on clinical suspicion as soon as blood cultures have been taken (only one set of cultures is needed). Some cases are complicated by endotoxic shock. The management of this condition is concerned with the maintenance of blood pressure, cardiac output and renal function, and much less with antimicrobial chemotherapy. Since the endotoxin is present in both living and dead bacterial cells, it is not important whether bactericidal or bacteristatic antibiotics are used. The position of corticosteroids in drug treatment of endotoxic shock is not clearly established, but if they are to be used, they should be given in gram quantities and not in the usual steroid replacement dosage.

Infective endocarditis is a specialized problem. Diagnosis is by isolation of the causative organism from blood cultures. Sets of blood cultures should be taken at three separate times when the patient's temperature is raised. Taking more sets of cultures increases the yield of positive cultures only very marginally. It is usually possible to wait for the results of the cultures and of antibiotic sensitivity tests before starting treatment. If the organism is fully sensitive to a single bactericidal antibiotic then adequate dosage of that drug should be given. If the organism is only partially sensitive to drugs tested, a combination of drugs may be needed, as routinely happens with infective endocarditis caused by enterococci. The laboratory should then test pairs of antibiotics against the pathogen *in vitro* ('chequer-board' studies) looking for evidence of bactericidal synergy. When a suitable pair of drugs has been found (very commonly penicillin and an aminoglycoside) these should be given to the patient in adequate dosage. The large majority of cases of infective endocarditis are caused by *Streptococcus viridans* which is usually sensitive to penicillin, and only 10% or so of cases are caused by enterococci. Because of this, if treatment must be started as soon as the blood cultures have been collected, I prefer that penicillin alone be given, retaining the possibility of adding an aminoglycoside antibiotic (usually gentamicin) later, if the cultures show this to be necessary. Others whose judgement I generally trust, prefer to give penicillin and an aminoglycoside drug at once and withdraw the second drug if it is shown to be unnecessary. There is no dispute, how-ever, on the point that only bactericidal antibiotics should be used in the treatment of infective endocarditis. When drug treatment of this condition is well established, its adequacy should be tested by measur-ing the peak concentration of the drug in the patient's blood. This should be at least 8 times the bactericidal concentration for the patient's pathogen (say, 4 times at mid-dose interval). If oral chemo-therapy is substituted for parenteral treatment, this 'back titration' of the patient's blood against his pathogen should be repeated. In patients receiving aminoglycoside antibiotics for this or any other infection, assays of the drug concentration in the blood should be performed in an attempt to regulate the dosage so as to minimize drug toxicity. The diagnosis and management of infective endocarditis requires the closest co-operation between clinicians and laboratory specialists.

There is much clinical confusion and misunderstanding about the importance of organisms circulating in the bloodstream of infected patients, or of patients thought to be infected. This is mostly due to a failure on the part of clinicians to ask whether the presence of the organisms is a manifestation of bacteraemia or of septicaemia. The dis-tinction is important: bacteraemia is probably a frequent event in both health and disease, and can be demonstrated to follow clinically insig-nificant activities such as brushing the teeth or chewing hard. The number of organisms circulating in the blood is probably not large, and their pathogenic significance is negligible. The situation in septicaemia is different: the number of organisms is large, they may replicate in the bloodstream and their presence gives rise to fever, rigors or even shock. Septicaemic patients are *ill*, and do not merely show a small rise in body temperature. Failure to draw a distinction between the two states leads to clinicians treating febrile patients as if they were about to succumb to rapidly fatal infection.

This clinical difficulty is well exemplified by the problems arising in the immune deficient hospital patient. Patients with impaired immun-ity caused by their disease (e.g. leukaemia) or by treatment (e.g. cortico-steroid drugs, irradiation, immunosuppressive therapy) are common in medical wards of hospitals in prosperous countries. Medical concern for the likelihood of infection in such patients is very natural. If a patient with, say, leukaemia with granulocytopenia (caused either by the disease or its treatment) dies, it is very likely to be because of infection. The managerial problem arises because a raised temperature in such patients is very common, much more so than infection. Should every such patient with a fever be treated as if he had septicaemia? I believe that this would be a mistake. Patients who look seriously ill and who develop a high fever with rigors, should be treated for presumed septicaemia, others not.

Many regimens have been developed for protecting immune deficient patients from infection, ranging from full protective isolation in a laminar flow environment with sterilized food and drink and no-touch nursing, through cubicle isolation combined with multiple antibiotic prophylaxis, to much more modest measures. At University College Hospital, the practice has been to give prophylactic co-trimoxazole, and this has been very successful in preventing intercurrent bacterial infection, although some viral or fungal infections do occur (Grüneberg et al., 1970). So successful has co-trimoxazole prophylaxis been in patients with leukaemia and agranulocytosis, that once the neutrophil count has risen above $1000/mm^3$ such patients are routinely managed in the open ward without additional measures to minimize the chance of infection. There are probably two reasons why co-trimoxazole works so well in such situations: the first is the maintained high level of sensitivity of hospital pathogens to the drug (as shown in Table 3), and the second is the marked reduction, in patients treated with co-trimoxazole, of the number of aerobic bacteria in the faecal flora and so, of the chance of endogenous infection. This method of preventing intercurrent infection is appreciated by the patient, his relatives and the attending staff, and is much cheaper than the alternatives. Clinical experience has shown that intercurrent bacterial infection in patients treated in this way is very rare. If septicaemia is suspected, other drugs such as chloramphenicol or, in the last resort, combinations including aminoglycoside antibiotics, are still available.

Pressure to prescribe antibiotics on the assumption that febrile patients may have septicaemia occurs in many departments of our hospitals. The clinical circumstances should be carefully considered and over reaction by the attending medical staff discouraged. Drug choice should be regulated such that the therapeutic response to clinical infection is carefully graded to fit the severity of the problem. If the most potent drug or combination of drugs is routinely used, what should the doctor do as an encore, if his infected patient's condition does not improve, or if it worsens?

The worst dilemmas arise with infections occurring in patients whose clinical state is parlous for other reasons. Every effort should be made to diagnose the infection precisely, so that the correct antibiotic treatment can be given. If this is not possible, then a drug (or combination of drugs) must be chosen which is likely to cover most eventualities. As already described (Chapter 4), a daily ward round by clinical microbiologists may be of value here. In the intensive care unit, one function of the microbiologist will be to try to restrain the clinician from using routinely drugs which should be used only in the last resort for treating life threatening infections. In the neonatal intensive care unit, it is often so difficult to make a diagnosis of the nature of infection, and events may move so rapidly, that the use of penicillin plus gentamicin is, sadly, almost routine for babies whose condition suddenly deteriorates. It may be that the recent introduction of mezlocillin and mecillinam may permit a reappraisal of the use of gentamicin in neonatal infections.

Wound infections

There is enormous variety in the location, severity, causative organisms and management of wound infections. The commonest pathogen is still *Staphylococcus aureus*, followed by *Streptococcus haemolyticus*, various coliform organisms and anaerobes. Mixed infections are common. In hospital, careful bacteriological studies are nearly always possible and the results of these should guide treatment. As already mentioned, the laboratory reports should be carefully assessed in the light of clinical circumstances in order to avoid vigorous treatment of harmless commensal organisms which may be only colonizing a lesion and not causing infection.

The scope of antibiotic treatment of infected wounds should be modest. The surgeon should always ask himself what result he is hoping for and then consider to what extent antibiotics will help. Closed abscesses will not often be sterilized by antibiotics. Draining abscesses will not benefit from antibiotic use. Antibiotics may be used to prevent the spread of bacteria locally through the tissues (cellulitis) or distantly by bloodstream spread. Additionally, they may have a place in the treatment of healing surgical wounds which become infected, since local sepsis will delay or prevent wound healing. When wound abscesses develop, they should be drained, since antibiotics will not help. When infection occurs in a surgical wound containing a haematoma, this also should be drained, since antibiotics are unlikely to penetrate to the site of infection in adequate concentration. Infected surgical wounds containing prostheses or other surgical aids such as metal pins or plates can rarely be sterilized by the use of antibiotics until the foreign body has been removed. When the removal of such an object is necessary, it should be done sooner rather than later, to give the patient the maximum benefit from antimicrobial chemotherapy before much granulation tissue, impenetrable to antibiotics, has been laid down. Prophylactic use of antibiotics in surgery should be confined to situations in which it has been shown to work, such as the prevention of gas gangrene in amputations of the lower limb under-taken because of vascular insufficiency. Prophylaxis should not be used in situations in which infection would be disastrous merely for that reason, unless it has been demonstrated clinically that the prophy-laxis proposed is effective.

Urinary tract infections

Most problems relating to UTI in hospital patients apply equally to similar infections seen in domiciliary practice (Chapter 5). The specific difficulties relate either to the choice of antibiotics or to the problem of catheter-associated infection.

The organisms causing UTI in hospital are somewhat different from those causing domiciliary infections. There are fewer infections caused by *Escherichia coli* and *Staphylococcus albus* (including micrococci) and more caused by *Klebsiella* spp., *Enterobacter* spp. and *Pseudo-monas aeruginosa*. Both because of the different mixture of species causing hospital UTI and because there is more antibiotic resistance among hospital isolates of normally sensitive species, the hospital urinary flora is more insensitive to the usual antibiotics than is the general practice urinary flora (Table 3). The ranking of antibiotics for use in 'blind' treatment is also different (Table 6). The practice of treating UTI on a 'best guess' basis in hospital can be condoned only occasionally (on grounds of clinical urgency) because it is so much easier to obtain urine culture results in hospital than in general practice, and because resistant pathogens are so much more common. Even when appropriate chemotherapy is given, the cure rate in hospital UTI will only be in the range of 60—70%, compared with the much higher cure rates (80—85%) to be expected with short course treatment of UTI in general practice. This is a reflection of the more complicated problems seen in hospital, where there is an adverse age structure among the patients treated, and where there are more people with recurrent UTI and with structural and functional abnormalities of the urinary tract (such as renal stones, tumours, prostatic enlargement and bladder diverticulae) which complicate treatment and affect its outcome. Antibiotics should be given in appropriate dosage for five to seven days, and tests of cure made in the usual way (Chapter 5). Drug choice should be made when the antibacterial sensitivities of the urinary pathogen are known. Reference to Table 3 shows that the choice will most often be between co-trimoxazole, nalidixic acid, trimethoprim and nitrofurantoin. On grounds of patient acceptability and likelihood of side effects, I would generally prefer co-trimoxazole under these circumstances. Incidentally, drug cost will be less of a factor in treatment choice in hospital than in general practice where it constitutes a large percentage of the total cost of medical care. In hospital, where a bed may cost £100 per day, if it can be shown that a more expensive drug results in more rapid cure than a cheaper one, the saving in bed costs would far outweigh the excess drug cost. Evidence of more rapid cure by one drug or another is, however, almost entirely lacking.

The second problem of UTI in hospitals is that of catheter-associated infection. It is well known that catheterization is associated with infection of the urinary tract. Insertion of an urethral catheter will cause UTI in 1—6% of uninfected patients. For this reason, it is no longer acceptable to pass a catheter for the sole purpose of collecting diagnostic samples or urine. It is also well recognized that passing a catheter into an infected urinary tract may cause the urinary organism to spill over into the bloodstream and even, upon occasion, cause endotoxic shock. The more usual problems, however, are caused by catheters which are left in position for lengthy periods. Much has been written about catheter hygiene, and the lesson of the importance of closed drainage systems for indwelling catheters has been well learnt.

Despite all precautions, however, catheters left in position for more than a few days give rise to an ascending UTI, the organism reaching the bladder not through the lumen of the catheter, but along the layer of mucopus between the urethra and the outside of the catheter. Antibiotic prophylaxis will not prevent this, and should not be attempted because it will merely ensure that when an infection is established, it will be caused by an organism resistant to the antibiotic given. In the presence of a catheter, only UTI which causes symptoms in the patient should be treated. Antibiotic treatment of UTI is disappointing, resulting either in failure or in only temporary success, with the original pathogen being rapidly replaced with another, usually more antibiotic resistant, organism. If prophylaxis or treatment must be attempted in the presence of an indwelling catheter, hexamine mandelate may be given, or the use of bladder washouts with noxythiolin may be attempted. In some cases, indwelling catheters are needed for a period and can later be removed, as after prostatectomy, for instance. A catheter-associated UTI may then resolve spontaneously without recourse to antimicrobial chemotherapy.

7

Control of infection in the community

Nay, one of the most eminent physicians, who has since published in Latin an account of those times, and of his observations, says that in one week there died twelve thousand people, and that particularly there died four thousand in one night.

. . . . . .

It is true that, as several physicians told my Lord Mayor, the fury of the contagion was such at some particular times, and people sickened so fast and died so soon, that it was impossible, and indeed to no purpose, to go about to inquire who was sick and who was well, or to shut them up with such exactness as the thing required, almost every house in a whole street being infected, and in many places every person in some of the houses; and that which was still worse, by the time that the houses were known to be infected, most of the persons known to be infected would be stone dead, and the rest run away for fear of being shut up;

A Journal of the Plague Year, Daniel Defoe (1661—1731)

Enormous changes have been brought about in society by the reduction of morbidity and mortality caused by infectious diseases. The nature of the change is borne in upon people from prosperous countries when they visit countries in the Third World and witness the impact of sporadic infections or of epidemics of infection caused by organisms long forgotten elsewhere. Readers of the diary of Samuel Pepys are struck by the frequency of the sudden death of relatively prosperous middle-aged people of his acquaintance in seventeenth century London caused by infections of various sorts, even in non-plague years. Pepys' account of the Great Plague of London in 1665, or Defoe's *Journal of the Plague Year*, are incomparable testimony to the transformation which has taken place.

These changes were not all brought about simultaneously, and even in the more fortunate countries, the process of control of infection is by no means complete. People are slow to grasp the fact that life has changed its character because of the removal of the threat of untimely death caused by infection. It is no longer necessary to produce large families in the hope that one or two of the children will survive, since most will now do so. The slowness of the realization of this change has resulted in enormous increases in human populations with the consequent overcrowding and malnutrition threatening to nullify the gains made.

Some of this transformation has been achieved as a result of better understanding of the nature of communicable diseases, following the work of the early microbiologists led by Pasteur and Koch. Probably, much greater benefits have flowed through social change pioneered by reformers without special medical knowledge. Some of the crucial developments were the provision of pure water, adequate sewage disposal and better nutrition; the reduction of overcrowding as better housing was introduced, and the change in attitudes to personal hygiene brought about at the beginning of the nineteenth century.

Water and sewage

'Pray to the Saints you may niver see cholera in a throop-thrain! 'Tis like the judgmint av God hittin' down from the nakid sky! . . . Thin the day began wid the noise in the carr'ges an' the rattle av the men on the platform fallin' over, arms an' all, as they stud for to answer the Comp'ny muster roll before goin' over to the camp. 'Tisn't for me to say what like the cholera was like. May be the Doctor cud ha' tould, av he hadn't dropped on to the platform from the door av a carriage where we was takin' out the dead. He died wid the rest. Some bhoys had died in the night. We tuk out siven, and twenty more was sickenin' as we tuk thim. The women was huddled up anyways, screamin' wid fear.'

> *The Daughter of the Regiment*, from *Plain Tales from the Hills.*
> Rudyard Kipling (1865–1936)

The provision of uncontaminated water supplies in the great cities of Europe is an event of the utmost importance. It began in the middle of the nineteenth century, and has brought to an end the great scourges of cholera and typhoid fever which used to decimate the urban populations from time to time. The significance of water supply in this group of infections was neatly demonstrated by the episode of the Broad Street pump. Dr J. Snow (a member of staff at University College Hospital) noticed that an outbreak of cholera in London was centred on this pump, and that those who drank water from it succumbed to the disease. He removed the handle of the pump so that water could no longer be drawn from it, and the cholera outbreak ceased.

The problem with water supply is to maintain it free of contamination by those bacteria, derived from sewage containing faecal material, which are capable of causing intestinal infections. In order to achieve this, sewage must be properly disposed of, and be kept separate from the water supply. Drinking water is subjected to processes of filtration and chlorination to control the numbers and types of bacteria present. The water supply industry undertakes stringent quality control of its product, and checks are also made by public health laboratories.

The satisfactory control of sewage in Western cities is again a relatively recent event. The skill of the Romans as sanitary engineers was lost during the dark ages. For centuries, the sewage of cities ran down open gutters in the streets, to find its way into a rudimentary system of underground sewers and so into the rivers from which water supplies were drawn. The population of Elizabethan London is said, as a consequence, to have suffered from chronic diarrhoea, largely due to bacillary dysentery. The great expansion of the population of London in the eighteenth and nineteenth centuries grossly overburdened the system. A new system of underground sewers lined with glazed earthenware was installed, and was widely copied elsewhere. It was eventually decided that the outflow of sewage systems could not just be released untreated into rivers and treatment in sewage farms was introduced. This treatment is aimed at the reduction in numbers of enteric pathogens by exposure to drying and to chemical action. Not all sewage is so treated: in many places untreated sewage is ducted out to sea, an unsavoury and unsatisfactory practice. The use of domestic

water closets began to be widespread in Western cities only at the end
of the last century.

Other water treatment problems include the purification of river
water, and of water in public swimming baths. The drainage of
swamps and marshes to remove standing water in which malarial
mosquitoes may breed is another important step in infection prevention in endemic areas.

The provision of pure water supplies and the safe removal of sewage
require considerable social organization. In times of war, earthquake
or other natural disaster, or even as a result of strikes by key workers,
these services are easily disrupted giving rise to fear of epidemics.

Food supply and waste disposal

> The hungry sheep look up, and are not fed,
> But, swoln with wind and the rank mist they draw,
> Rot inwardly and foul contagion spread.

Lycidas, John Milton (1608—1674)

At every stage of food production, preparation, storage, distribution,
sale and cooking, infectious hazards may arise. Livestock should be
kept as free of parasites as possible, a joint task for farmers and veterinary workers. Some successes have been the establishment of tuberculosis free herds of cattle, and the gradual eradication of brucellosis.
New problems arise from intensive farming methods, such as the
occurrence of antibiotic resistant *Salmonella* spp. colonizing livestock
given antibiotics in their feed to promote more rapid growth. At the
slaughterhouse, great care is taken to avoid contamination of
carcasses, and these are inspected by veterinary workers and food
inspectors looking for evidence of parasitic diseases transmissible to
man (e.g. tapeworms or *Trichinella spiralis* infection). Meat must be
stored in a cool place or be refrigerated, away from flies or rats or other
disease carrying vectors, until processed or sold. Ceaseless attention to
detail is necessary to prevent tragedy. A single lapse in a salmon
cannery in Alaska resulted in cases of botulism in England in 1978. In
1964, a consignment of canned corned beef was contaminated with
river water containing *Salmonella typhi* in Argentina. Later, the
contents of a large tin were sliced up in a shop in Aberdeen giving rise

to several hundred cases of typhoid fever. The quality control activities of big food firms are very exacting and serious lapses are rare. Foodstuffs on sale in shops and markets are randomly tested by the public health and market authorities. Some foodstuffs are the subject of special attention, examples being the pasteurization or sterilization of milk, and the testing of ice-cream or shellfish.

The removal of domestic waste is a matter of public health concern. If left to stand, it smells unpleasant, and more importantly, provides an opportunity for the multiplication of flies, mice and rats, any of which may carry disease. Local authorities do all in their power to control the numbers of such pests. Public health inspectors inspect commercial food storage facilities and the kitchens of restaurants partly to check on hygienic standards and partly to see that pests are controlled.

At times of social upheaval, these measures may easily be disrupted, so that governments need to have contingency plans ready for the public protection.

Surveillance of infection

> One sickly sheep infects the flock,
> And poisons all the rest.
>
> *Against Evil Company, Divine Songs for Children* xxi.
> Isaac Watts (1674—1748)

In different countries, the surveillance of infection is undertaken in different ways. Two types of reporting are usual, however, the notification of various clinical infections to the relevant public health authorities by doctors attending patients, and the notification of laboratory isolations of certain pathogens to central epidemiological offices.

Most countries require the notification of certain clinical infections, which differ from time to time and between countries, making this a statutory duty of the doctor. The method is subject to clinical diagnostic error, and to gross under reporting by doctors who may be ignorant of their legal duty or who cannot be bothered to make a report. Nonetheless, some crude data of epidemiological interest may be obtained, which may draw attention to changes in the pattern of infection. Sometimes, the pattern of notification may serve as a reminder of the need to bolster the immunity of susceptible individuals by immunization programmes.

Of much greater value is the system whereby diagnostic laboratories, public health laboratories and reference laboratories report microbial isolates from clinical material to central national bureaux. These reports are much more reliable than are clinical notifications and may provide more useful evidence on which to base national infection control programmes. In the United Kingdom, the Communicable Diseases Reference Centre at Colindale collates the laboratory information which it receives and publishes weekly and quarterly Communicable Disease Reports which go to all public health authorities and clinical laboratories in the country. The information in these reports keeps clinical microbiologists in touch with the pattern of infections seen elsewhere in the country, an invaluable service. Other countries have similar infection surveillance centres, all of which provide information for the World Health Organization. The speed of communication of such findings worldwide is such that the international spread of infections can be anticipated long before it happens. An example of this is the worldwide watch for the emergence of new antigenic types of influenza virus. When these are detected, there may be enough time for new protective immunizations to be developed before the virus has spread far.

Containment of infection

> This other Eden, demi-paradise,
> This fortress built by Nature for herself,
> Against infection and the hand of war.

Richard II, Act II, Sc. 1, Q. 40, William Shakespeare (1564—1616)

When certain diagnoses of infectious disease are made, the attending clinician may have to consider what steps should be taken to minimize the spread of contagion. Sometimes such decisions are taken jointly with public health officials, and sometimes they are matters of national policy. In this way, children with measles or chickenpox are kept away from others thought to be susceptible. Patients with rubella are kept away from women in the early stages of pregnancy in order to avoid the risk of affecting the foetus. (Before rubella vaccination was available, it used to be the custom in some circles to arrange 'rubella parties' at which, it was hoped, a child with german measles would pass it on to others who had not yet had the disease.)

In some cases of communicable disease, hospitalization may be required, and decisions will then have to be taken as to whether the patient should be nursed in the open ward or in a cubicle, with or without special nursing precautions (barrier nursing). In some infections, spread is so likely that admission to an ordinary hospital is not appropriate, and such patients are sent to infectious diseases units. This may also be appropriate in some other infections on grounds of public anxiety.

Decisions of this sort are initially taken by the attending doctor, but in cases of doubt, advice may be sought from local microbiologists or from the public health authorities. The latter will clearly opt for isolation in special units for patients with smallpox, Lassa fever, viral haemorrhagic diseases, plague and the like. Quite modest precautions will contain the infective hazards of enteric fever or hepatitis. Many infections are contagious only for a brief time, after which relaxation of isolation procedures is appropriate. Specialized knowledge is required to decide when this should be done for each disease. There is no direct relationship between the severity of infectious diseases and their infectivity.

In some cases, governments have passed legislation or made regulations controlling certain diseases. Examples of this in the United Kingdom include forbidding the importation of any mammal capable of carrying rabies without appropriate quarantine, and the requirement to slaughter livestock suffering from anthrax where they are, the carcasses being buried on the spot.

A very important function of public health workers is the following-up of contacts of certain infectious diseases. This may, upon occasion, involve the contacting of thousands of people as happens sometimes with outbreaks of enteric fever in countries in which it is not endemic, and as used to happen following the identification of cases of smallpox in Europe. Where enteric fever is spread by catering workers, there may be considerable problems, as exemplified by the case of 'Typhoid Mary', a cook who caused a series of outbreaks of typhoid fever around New York at the beginning of this century. The difficulties are enhanced by public anxieties, pandered to by the news media. In the Aberdeen typhoid outbreak of 1964 there were more than 500 cases, but only a couple of deaths, and those in people already very ill for other reasons. The investigation of outbreaks of this sort involves the search for cases and for carriers, with a view to their prompt treatment and avoidance of further cycles of food-borne infection. This may require the deployment of considerable laboratory resources. With other diseases, contacts may be sought in order that they may be offered immunization, or be kept under observation.

A different type of contact tracing is undertaken in relation to venereal diseases. The object here is to arrange for effective treatment of unsuspecting sufferers from syphilis or gonorrhoea, and by so doing to prevent further spead of infection. This work is usually undertaken by specialized staff, working from venereology clinics, who are trained in the techniques of obtaining sensitive information and of approaching contacts with great tact. The maintenance of clinical confidence is very important in this area. In some enlightened countries (not including the United Kingdom), prostitutes must be licensed and are regularly checked for freedom from infection.

A corollary of contact tracing by public health workers or others is that there must be adequate support, not only by laboratories capable of providing rapid diagnosis, but also by clinics capable of dealing with immunization, surveillance or treatment, according to need. Much of this provision will be unnecessary most of the time, but it must be available on a standby basis for the occasions when it is required.

Immunization

Thou shalt not be afraid for any terror by night: nor for the arrow that flieth by day.

For the pestilence that walketh in darkness: nor for the sickness that destroy-eth in the noon-day.

A thousand shall fall beside thee, and ten thousand at thy right hand: but it shall not come nigh thee.

Psalms xci. 5

Immunization is an area of infection prevention which has, almost uniquely, followed hard on the heels of advances in knowledge brought about by microbiological research. Many infectious diseases which were formerly scourges of mankind have become rarities among populations in which immunization is common.

Perhaps the most striking single example of this is the worldwide eradication of smallpox now claimed by the World Health Organization, in which immunization (vaccination) played a large part. Smallpox is an unusual disease in that it is caused by only one type of pathogen, the variola virus, which apparently has no host other than man. Another feature is that man either has the infection or he does not: there is no carrier state. Jenner's pioneering work (done without microbiological knowledge) in the protection of those who are susceptible to variola (i.e. all those who have not had the infection) by immunization with fluid from cow pox lesions, led to campaigns of mass vaccination of populations. As a result, smallpox died out in the prosperous societies which had been immunized, except for occasional outbreaks following sporadic importation of the disease from endemic areas abroad where the population had not been protected. In the nineteen seventies, the World Health Organization led a campaign in the countries in which smallpox was still endemic aimed at its final eradication. Cases were identified and isolated, and all contacts were vaccinated. Local populations were motivated to report cases, the number of which reduced rapidly. First one country and then another was declared free of the disease, until it now looks as if the campaign may have eradicated smallpox worldwide. If this proves to be the case, and there may still be some scope for uncertainty, it will be an unique achievement. Meanwhile, there seems to be no medical reason to continue smallpox vaccination, except for virologists working in laboratories still holding stocks of the virus. (It is ironic that what may prove to be the last case of this disease occurred in Britain, where the infection was not endemic, as a result of a laboratory accident.)

Not all immunization programmes have been as successful as that against smallpox. Some have been successful in controlling infections which have then become rare in immunized populations, leading to people forgetting the nature of the threat and failing to maintain immunization programmes. An example of this is immunization against diphtheria, one of the great killers of children in prosperous societies before the Second World War. Diphtheria has become exceedingly rare in immunized societies, and a whole new generation has grown up to whom the disease does not seem a reality, with the result that the acceptance rate of immunization has fallen alarmingly. This fall has been paralleled by similar falls in acceptance levels for other immunizations of proved effectiveness such as those against tetanus and poliomyelitis. The problem of reduced uptake of immunizations has been in the United Kingdom made more severe by public concern about whooping cough immunization.

Whooping cough is a clinical entity, many cases of which are caused by infection with the bacterium *Bordetella pertussis*. Within that species, there are a number of serotypes which occur with differing prevalence from time to time and from place to place. Immunization can, for technical reasons, be protective against only a selection of the more prevalent serotypes of *B. pertussis* rather than against all strains, and has no protective effect against other causative agents of whooping cough such as adenovirus infection. Recently there has been public anxiety about the neurological damage occasionally caused in children by whooping cough immunization. Unfortunately, the 'experts' were unduly authoritarian in their public assurances that neurological damage was not caused by *B. pertussis* immunization and that such immunization was highly protective. Independent assessment by uncommitted experts suggested that neither claim was true. The public lost faith in expert opinion and the uptake of *B. pertussis* immunization fell. This led to the fall in the uptake of other immunizations commonly linked with it, i.e. tetanus, diphtheria and poliomyelitis. This is a tragedy because, whatever the situation with *B. pertussis*, these other immunizations are both safe and effective. A more becoming humility on the part of the experts in admitting their relative ignorance of matters in which no one knew all the answers, might have maintained public confidence.

When all of the population is immune to a pathogen it can establish no foothold and the disease which it causes disappears. If the level of immunity in the population falls (because of poor uptake of immunization, for example) there will be a reduction in the so-called 'herd immunity' which protects against the disease becoming established again until a certain proportion of the population is once again susceptible. It seems that as long as about 60% of the population is immune, the disease does not establish itself. There is, therefore, a need on public health grounds to re-establish public confidence in safe, effective immunizations such as those against diphtheria, tetanus and poliomyelitis, in order to maintain herd immunity.

One problem here is to explain to clinicians and to the public what can be expected of immunization, and a second problem is to reconcile the ethical dilemma of doing things (for the best of motives) which, although designed to benefit society at large, may harm the individual. Not all immunizations are equally effective or equally safe. It is important to consider the chance of individuals acquiring the infection if unimmunized and the nature and severity of the disease if it is contracted. Each disease should be considered on its merits.

In the case of smallpox, the rare risk of vaccination damage was well worth running when the disease was prevalent because the vaccination was highly protective against a very contagious disease with a high death rate, and for which no effective treatment was available. The need to maintain immunity by repeat vaccination every few years did not seriously affect this assessment. Now that the disease has apparently been eradicated, continued smallpox vaccination of populations would be irresponsible. Similarly, in areas in which yellow fever is endemic, immunization against the disease should always be undertaken, because infection is highly likely and often fatal, there being no specific treatment for it, and because specific immunization is highly protective, conferring lifelong immunity at small risk.

The other extreme is exemplified by cholera immunization for those living in or visiting endemic areas. Although cholera prophylaxis is not associated with much risk, it requires an initial series of injections followed by booster injections every six months. The level of protection against infection is not high, it being hoped rather that the severity of infection will be diminished, and the chance of infection is not great except during an outbreak. Although death rates from infection used to be high, effective treatment is now available and death rates should be low. The case for cholera prophylaxis therefore appears to me to be relatively weak. Immunization of populations living around the centre of an outbreak of the disease may be useful in attempting to create a *cordon sanitaire*, but even this has been questioned.

Immunization against typhoid and paratyphoid fevers by the use of

TAB vaccine has been available for many years. Here, too, the value of the procedure may be questioned. The injections must be given as a series initially, followed by boosters at regular, short intervals and may produce local reactions at the site of injection and a systemic upset. It seems that the antigens of paratyphoid A and B bacilli are responsible for most of the trouble and, in any case, do not provide much protection against paratyphoid fever. The typhoid antigens cause less upset on injection, do provide partial protection, and lead to milder, modified, typhoid fever in those who contract the disease despite immunization. The risk of acquiring such infections should be borne in mind when considering whether to offer the immunization. Enteric fever is a very disagreeable disease, but effective treatment in the form of chloramphenicol or co-trimoxazole does exist. All things considered, I am not very convinced of the value of TAB immunization. If it is felt desirable to offer immunization in individual circumstances, this should be given against typhoid fever alone, and attempts should not be made to protect against paratyphoid fever at the same time.

Opinions differ as to the desirability of attempting the prevention of viral hepatitis (type A) in susceptible people by the use of injections of immune globulin. This is a passive immunization lasting only as long as the injected antibodies circulate in the recipient, usually only for a matter of weeks. It may be sensible to try such immunization in patients who are ill for some other reason and who come in contact with infectious cases of viral hepatitis A. The case for routine prophylaxis of travellers repeatedly travelling to areas in which the disease is endemic is much weaker because of the short lived protection offered, this becoming shorter and shorter with successive injections.

In recent years, rubella vaccination has been widely introduced. Its uptake is not dictated by any desire to prevent what is generally a very mild or even subclinical infection. It is offered to pubertal girls in an attempt to ensure that if they later become pregnant they will be immune to the disease and so not be at risk of producing rubella affected babies if exposed to infection in the first four months of pregnancy. This laudable aim is made difficult to attain by ethical problems. Is it reasonable to expose a population of girls to a small (but finite) risk in order to protect a population of babies not yet born, conceived, or even contemplated? Since many of the girls will already be immune to rubella by previous (often undiagnosed) infection, is it reasonable to give them prophylaxis which they do not require? Since the vaccine used is a living rubella virus which will be shed by those receiving it, what of the possibility of its leading to infection of women in early pregnancy, and so to the causation of just that foetal damage which it is desired to prevent? Once successive cohorts of the female population have been immunized for a sufficient number of years, the problem of rubella affected foetuses is expected to disappear, but the (in this case, small) problem of vaccine damage will remain. Looking at the problem overall, I am sure that routine rubella vaccination is a wise policy, but I have a continuing unease about what to say to the parents of the very few vaccine damaged children, immunized not for their own benefit, but for that of others. I wish to make it clear that I disapprove of giving immunization to those who are already immune, when a simple blood test for rubella antibodies could show this.

Vaccination against measles (morbilli) presents other problems. Measles is an unpleasant infection contracted in childhood by nearly everyone. Infected children are miserable and fretful for a week, and may suffer a variety of rare complications of the associated viraemia. Most complications following measles are due to secondary bacterial invasion and include otitis media, acute bronchitis, broncho-pneumonia, pulmonary atelectasis and bronchiectasis. The idea of preventing such complications is attractive. Again, a live virus is used, and this produces a modified attack of measles. In my experience, this is often only marginally milder than the disease produced by wild strains. A more theoretical problem is posed by the fact that, since measles immunization is a relatively recent introduction, it is not yet known how long the immunity to infection lasts. If the effect of measles immunization in childhood were only to postpone naturally occurring infection until adult life, when measles is a much more serious disease, the overall effect would be harmful. More evidence of benefit is needed here.

Influenza immunization is an enormous subject because it depends for its effect on being directed against the prevalent antigenic types of influenza virus. The influenza viruses have an amazing capacity to generate new antigenic variants. Some of these prove to be sufficiently different from previous serotypes for their spread to find populations of human beings susceptible to infection with them. There has arisen a worldwide network of laboratories examining isolates of influenza virus for serological variation and plotting the spread of influenza. Interestingly, waves of infection with new serotypes of influenza viruses seem often to originate in China and to spread from there. New types are given scientific names describing their date and site of first isolation and their antigenic makeup. The news media seem anxious to accord the new pathogens a more frightening description and christen them 'Chinese 'flu', 'Hong Kong 'flu' or 'Red 'flu'. This generates public fear, often quite unreasonably since many of these pathogens do not spread far, and may occasion little serious infection. Politicians may get in on the act, seeking public approval by dynamic action. A particularly unfortunate example occurred in the United States of America some years ago, when the President committed the government to ensuring that the entire population be immunized against the so-named 'Swine 'flu'. This strain had been isolated from some soldiers in Fort Worth, Texas, but showed little propensity to spread, and caused little serious disease because of antigenic relationships to previous serotypes. Enormous expense must have been incurred, and lives lost, in the reaction against an unreal threat, with consequent loss of public confidence in the advice given.

The drug industry has an extraordinary capacity to develop, very rapidly, vaccines against new serotypes of influenza virus as they arise and show a propensity to spread. The selection and use of such vaccines requires balanced judgement. Most waves of influenza cause infections which are dangerous predominantly to patients with pre-existing heart or lung disease. Such patients should be offered influenza vaccination every autumn to cover them over the high risk, winter season. Apart from that, epidemics of influenza may cause massive absenteeism from work because many employees are affected simultaneously by infections of modest severity. Employers may think it reasonable to offer influenza immunization to at least their key personnel in order that relatively normal services may be maintained. Occasionally, a more than usually virulent influenza outbreak may occur, such as that which followed the First World War. If that should happen it might be reasonable to attempt the mass immunization of whole populations. Such decisions should be taken dispassionately, a task which would be easier in the absence of media generated hysteria which is rarely justified by the facts.

Health education

Human history becomes more and more a race between education and catastrophe.

The Outline of History, Chapter 15, H. G. Wells (1866–1946)

Health education occupies a central position in the control of infection in a community. It is conducted in many ways, is aimed at various audiences, and is attended with differing degrees of success. Health education is aimed at professionals in the health industry through the agency of a wide range of different techniques. Since this is clearly entirely successful it will not be necessary to discuss it here. More scope is offered in discussion of the health education addressed to the person in the street.

Some health education reaches the public through posters hung in public places and conveying simple messages: 'Coughs and sneezes spread diseases', 'Now wash your hands' or 'Flies spread disease'. (The rôle of the educator is everywhere derided — I have seen the last of these mottoes amended: 'Flies spread disease — keep yours buttoned'.) In the same way, many public lavatories display notices giving information as to where help may be sought by those who think that they may have venereal infections.

We are exposed to advertising by commercial interests, and some of this is educational, although not always correct. Some of the least helpful is related to the domestic use of disinfectants. We are urged to pour disinfectant down the toilet, for reasons that are not clear to me. We are also told that 'X kills 99% of household germs', a useless objective, if true. If it merely means that X reduces a typical bacterial load from, say, 1 000 000/ml to 10 000/ml, where is the benefit (unless to those engaged in the production and sale of X)? Since there will never be any shortage of misguided, misleading and incorrect advice from commercial interests, it is a duty of health professionals and of consumer groups to right the balance. Medical columns in newspapers and periodicals may be very valuable in this way.

The education of specialist groups in the importance of correct procedures aimed at minimization of infection may be of great relevance. Thus, trainee veterinarians, farm workers, food handlers, catering staff and many others should receive instruction on relevant matters. This is shamefully neglected in most such groups in nearly all countries, leaving much scope for improved practice and reduced levels of infection.

Some of the most important advice to the public on infection prevention arrives in apparently irrelevant ways concerned with matters such as nutrition, housing, clothing and personal hygiene. There seems little doubt that well fed populations are less infection prone than the malnourished, although objective proof is often lacking and there is dissension as to the nature of a satisfactory diet. In prosperous societies, in which people are in the happy position of choosing what they will eat, there is a job to be done in educating them into appropriate choices. It is sometimes claimed that the population of Britain has never been as well fed as it was during the Second World War, when serious food shortages at home and the need to import the balance over submarine infested seas, led to the government introducing a rationing scheme which guaranteed enough (and little more) of a balanced diet for everyone. In more prosperous times, Britons have chosen more expensive, more convenient foods, and now eat too much and of the wrong things. It must be conceded, however, that greater British liability to infection is not apparent.

Housing standards have a bearing on the likelihood of infection. People must be educated into wanting light, well ventilated houses with sufficient space to avoid overcrowding. Governments and local authorities must be educated into requiring toilet facilities and adequate washing facilities to be installed in all homes. Running water must be available wherever food is prepared so that it can be cleaned and so that handwashing by those doing the cooking is encouraged. Suitable fly- and rodent-proof food stores should be available.

Clothing choice and care also have a bearing on infection. In mediaeval times, people in Europe wore woollen clothes which were warm and durable, but which were difficult to keep clean. At the time, people scarcely washed, and so their clothes stank and became filthy and verminous. Scent and herbs were used to mask the stench. When the cotton trade was established in the eighteenth century it became possible for the first time for ordinary people to have cheap, light, easily washed undergarments. Personal cleanliness began to be fashionable again among the upper classes for the first time since the fall of the Roman Empire in the west. This changed attitude to personal hygiene was given added impetus by the large number of men forced into naval service in the Napoleonic wars, since the discipline of shipboard life imposed by gentlemen officers required bodily cleanliness. This, and the large number of lower class servants working in the houses of the well-to-do in the nineteenth century, resulted in a social revolution, personal cleanliness (if not next to godliness) at least being regarded as a requirement of decent living. (It may be noted that many people living in hot eastern countries still regard westerners as being deficient in personal hygiene.) The new bodily cleanliness and the more frequent changing and washing of clothes virtually brought about the end of vermin infestation and with it the disappearance of plague and typhus. These gains need to be maintained by public education through advertising, newspapers, radio and television.

Nowadays, the main means of communication are through advertising and the newspapers, and by the medium of radio and television broadcasting. Never has so much information been so readily communicated to so many. We are in a position to use these powerful tools of communication for the general benefit in passing on to the public information which will help to inculcate attitudes leading to the prevention of infection. This task is at present in the hands of communicators who know little of the problems. The main challenge to members of the medical profession here, is to learn communicative skills so that they can use the media themselves in order to pass on their knowledge. Alternatively, they should educate the professional communicators with regard to the true facts of infection and its prevention.

8

Control of infection
in hospitals

Incens'd with indignation Satan stood
Unterrifi'd and like a comet burn'd
That fires the length of Ophiucus huge
In th' arctic sky, and from his horrid hair
Shakes pestilence and war.

Paradise Lost, John Milton (1608—1674)

Infection in hospitals is part of the problem of infection in general. Hospitals import infection from the population outside and are lively exporters of bacteria to the community at large. My excuse for dealing with the prevention of infection in hospitals separately is that it presents special problems scarcely encountered in infection prevention elsewhere. Hospitals present such a combination of susceptible patients (and staff), virulent and transmissible pathogens, and means and opportunities of causing infection that it might be thought surprising that anyone escapes unharmed. To the extent that this is true there is some reason for modest pride in what has been achieved. Complacency is inappropriate: about 5 patients in every hundred admitted to 'acute' hospitals develop infections in hospital, and 3% of those are fatal. Another 10 patients in every 100 admitted to 'acute' hospitals will be infected on admission. The total amount of illness, misery and death caused by infections in hospital patients is enormous, and its economic significance is great. A recent estimate of

133

the direct and indirect costs of hospital-acquired infection in the U.S.A. put the figure at $2000 million per annum. To the extent that such infections are preventable (perhaps 50%) there is every reason to take the challenge seriously and to spare no effort in doing so.

In modern hospitals, the problem of infection prevention has been entrusted to Control of Infection Committees. These are chaired by the Control of Infection Officer who may be either a microbiologist or an interested clinician. He will be supported by nursing staff with a specialized training (control of infection nurses). Control of Infection Committees will have varying membership but may typically include: a physician, a surgeon, a paediatrician, an obstetrician, the local environmental health specialist, the head of the central sterile supply department and those of other allied units such as the theatre sterile supply unit and the medical equipment disinfection unit, a senior pharmacist, a supplies officer, the catering officer, the head of the domestic cleaning staff, a works officer, senior nurses in various departments, nurse teachers, control of infection nurses, and an administrator. Others may be co-opted from time to time. Such committees will produce an Infection Control Manual which will lay down safe procedures for a multitude of activities within the hospital. The committee will review local procedures continually and will keep the Infection Control Manual up to date in the light of changes in practice. Problems occurring anywhere in the hospital may be referred to the committee which should report to the authority responsible for the hospital. Agreed policies are binding on all staff until changes are agreed.

In the remainder of this chapter I propose to discuss briefly some of the innumerable topics which would be considered by a Control of Infection Committee. Although it will be obvious that many of these subjects are inter-related it is unavoidable that each be discussed separately.

Admission policy

No 'acute' hospital can refuse to admit patients with infection, but some degree of selection is usual. Most paediatric units are reluctant to admit children who may be suffering from the early, atypical stages of highly contagious infectious diseases spread by the respiratory route, such as measles and chickenpox, or from other conditions capable of rapid transmission to other patients (e.g. scarlet fever). Such patients will be referred to infectious diseases units for admission. Patients with a variety of other infections of varying degrees of transmissibility may or may not be admitted depending on local policy. Some units are content to nurse patients with enteric fever or infective hepatitis, others are not. Such decisions may depend upon nursing staff availability, the ability to undertake barrier nursing, the availability of single rooms and the susceptibility of other patients or staff to the infection. Each hospital will have to define its policy in relation to the admission of patients known to have open tuberculosis. No hospital other than those specifically designated for the purpose should knowingly admit patients suffering from smallpox, Lassa fever, Ebola fever, Marburg disease or other potentially lethal and highly infectious conditions.

Hospital design

Careful attention to the numerous features of hospital design may help to minimize the spread of infection. The most important of these is the avoidance of overcrowding of patients. The fewer patients in a ward and the greater the distance between them, the smaller the chance of infection. The ideal is the provision of a separate room for each patient, but this has disadvantages in loneliness of patients, less ready observation by ward staff, and a requirement for more nurses. None-theless, some cubicles should be available on every ward for infectious conditions which may arise and which do not justify removal else-where. These may alternatively be used for patients especially at risk from infection.

Proper ventilation should be borne in mind as a major design feature. In most parts of a hospital this merely means the provision of plentiful fresh air, but in some specialized areas such as operating theatres or the sterile production area of the pharmacy, it may involve positive pressure ventilation to ensure unidirectional air flow, or even so-called laminar air flow. The design of units requiring such facilities is a highly skilled undertaking, and expert advice should always be sought (but often is not). Central heating, humidification and air conditioning systems also have a bearing on infection prevention, and their design should be reviewed.

Operating theatres have, in the past, often been designed by those who work in them (surgeons and nurses) with scant regard to the need to build into them features which will reduce infection risks. They should be designed to ensure that 'clean' and 'dirty' procedures are totally separated. Sterile equipment should be assembled in a 'clean' area, taken to the patient, used and routed to a 'dirty' area to be despatched, for reprocessing. This means that there must be one way traffic through a theatre suite so that 'clean' and 'dirty' materials never cross in transit. The flow of filtered air must be carefully arranged to flow from 'clean' to 'dirty' areas and so to the exterior. This requires obsessional supervision in the use of the theatres, but if the basic design is faulty, even the most painstaking rituals will be ineffective. The days of amateur operating theatre design should have passed.

Design features in the wards such as the provision of adequate bathing, washing, and toilet facilities; of adequate waste disposal facilities, including drainage from bed pan washing machines, and of easily cleanable floor, ceiling and wall surfaces must all receive attention. The design of ward kitchens and their use for the production of beverages and snacks should be reviewed.

Those who design hospital buildings need expert advice on the infection prevention aspects of their work.

Infectious diseases

Hospitals should not knowingly admit cases of infectious diseases excluded by their admission policy. Nonetheless, it will often happen that infectious diseases occur in patients in the wards, either because the disease was not recognized at the time of admission or because of subsequent infection. Each of the infections which may occur should be separately listed in the Infection Control Manual with information on its causative organism, sources of infection, portals of entry, incubation period, period of communicability, and appropriate management in terms of isolation procedures and special precautions. Notification procedures should be defined for every type of infection. Internal notification will ensure that the control of infection staff in the hospital know about what is happening and can take suitable action. External notification to the relevant public health authorities will ensure that the wider community interest is protected. Most countries have lists of infections which must statutorily be notified, and steps should be taken to remind hospital staff of their legal duties in this respect.

Provision should be made by contingency planning for appropriate action to be taken when an emergency occurs in relation to infection, as may happen with the admission of unrecognized cases of smallpox or Lassa fever, for instance. An emergency committee should be constituted to take control in such eventualities, and its course of action should be defined ahead of need.

Isolation

Isolation procedures are of two kinds, those designated to prevent the spread of infection from one patient to others, and those intended to protect a susceptible patient from extraneous micro-organisms (protective isolation). Procedures for both situations should be carefully defined in the Infection Control Manual, and the materials needed should be available for rapid deployment as required. Ward staff must be carefully trained and supervised in carrying out the appropriate routines if these are to be effective.

The measures to be taken will depend upon the disease. Some infections may be safely managed on the open ward, others should be transferred to a separate room. Segregated patients may need 'barrier nursing' to prevent the spread of organisms, or they may need full isolation in a specialized infectious diseases unit. Each condition should be listed in the Infection Control Manual and the degree of segregation appropriate indicated. This will depend upon the transmissibility of an infection and not on its severity. Thus infections such as tetanus or gas gangrene, although often serious, do not require segregation for infection control reasons because cross-infection is very improbable. Spread of some other infections is possible, but unlikely, in hospitals, provided normal procedures are carried out. An example of this is enteric fever which has often been nursed in general medical wards for some time, without spread to other people, before the diagnosis was made.

Different detailed procedures will be laid down in the Infection Control Manual for various conditions depending on the mode of spread of the infection concerned: whether by contact, by inhalation, or by ingestion. Procedures should be defined for cleaning rooms during occupation by infected patients and after their departure (terminal cleaning). Rarely, fumigation will be needed, and the procedure and indications for this should be covered. The cleaning or disinfection of medical equipment used in treatment of infected patients should be considered, as should the problems of waste disposal and laundry.

Upon occasion, it may be thought desirable to close a ward, a unit, or even a hospital because of some infectious problem. This should be done rarely, only by those well enough informed to judge its necessity, and with careful consideration of the problems raised. These problems will include the transfer of existing patients elsewhere, and the provision of alternative accommodation for new patients. Arrangements must be made to warn other units or hospitals which may have to cope with an unexpected, additional load. All clinicians and nursing staff affected must be informed of the decision at once, as must the hospital administration. The public health authorities should be alerted to the problem, and steps taken to answer enquiries from the press. Care must be taken to avoid panic among patients, relatives, staff and the population at large. Procedures governing such closures or reductions of service should be laid down in the Manual.

Simple precautions

One of the main means of spread of infection in hospital or outside, is by carriage of organisms on the hands. This leads to a need to insist on scrupulous handwashing in order to reduce the opportunities for transmission of infection. This will apply not only to the usual conventions of handwashing before handling food or after micturition or defaecation, but also to handwashing before and after a range of hospital procedures including various clinical examinations, setting up an intravenous drip and passing a catheter. Washing before the procedure helps to protect the patient on whom it is to be conducted, and washing afterwards protects other patients. The word 'convention' in relation to handwashing should not mean that it is performed in a slipshod or token manner, it is too important for that. The original observations by Semmelweiss in Vienna showed the cardinal importance of careful handwashing by medical staff in the prevention of the scourge of the obstetric wards, puerperal fever. The simple measures introduced by him largely prevented deaths due to what was almost certainly haemolytic streptococcal infection. Nowadays the main route of transmission of hospital infections caused by Gram-negative bacilli is on the hands of nursing and medical staff who take insufficient care with handwashing.

However thorough the process, and however powerful the soap or disinfectant used in handwashing, the main factor in reducing the bacterial load on the hands is the thoroughness of their subsequent drying. Bacteria are much more easily transferred on a moist surface than a dry one (hence the desirability of moistening a swab before sampling a dry surface).

Part of the basic routine of infection control is the attempt to prevent shedding of upper respiratory tract organisms by staff by the wearing of masks. These should only be worn when appropriate, should be worn over nose and mouth, and when worn, should be capable of fulfilling the function expected. The Infection Control Manual should give guidance on this.

The specification of gowns, aprons, white coats, and gloves, and the wearing of boots or overshoes by hospital staff should similarly be reviewed. Appropriate designs should be chosen. When and where they should be worn, and by whom, should be considered. Arrangements for changing should be adequate, so that potentially contaminated protective clothing is not taken around the wards, or into operating theatres or canteens. Laundry arrangements for such clothing should be made. Disposal routines should be well understood.

Special precautions

Pre-operative skin preparation is often a ritual in the wrong sense of the word, that is an ineffective, time consuming, wasteful procedure. Thorough washing and drying of the skin is as good as and cheaper than some established procedures. Shaving, washing and skin disinfectant procedures should be agreed and defined in the Manual.

Care of wounds, removal of stitches or surgical drains, and the changing of dressings should be undertaken with the utmost care. Such procedures should be performed in a room set aside for the purpose, if possible. If not, they should not be undertaken in the ward until the dust suspended in the air by such procedures as floor sweeping or bedmaking has had time to settle (about an hour). A no-touch technique should be used. Detailed procedures should be laid down in the Manual, and adhered to.

Urethral catheterization should be performed as a minor surgical procedure, in the right place, at the right time, and by trained staff using a no-touch technique. Procedures for this and for catheter hygiene, and policies for the frequency of catheter changes for patients needing indwelling catheters, should be described in the Manual. Some hospitals have set up catheter teams whose task it is to carry out these duties for all catheterized patients in the hospital.

The setting up of intravenous infusions is a skilled technique. It is also an excellent way of risking local or disseminated infection. The longer the infusion is left in position, the greater the risk. The use of central venous catheters (long lines) whether for monitoring purposes, for the administration of drugs, or for intravenous feeding, is a still greater hazard. Detailed policies for the insertion of lines, for their resiting and for their routine observation and care should be written into the Manual. There is much to be said for instituting an intravenous drip team in busy hospitals to take care of these procedures. Additional attention should be paid in the Manual to the practice of adding drugs to intravenous infusions. A system must be set up for checking fluids for intravenous infusion and for recognizing and investigating possible episodes of infusion fluid infection. Such policies require the skilled assistance of the pharmacy staff.

The pharmacy

Considering their potential for giving rise to outbreaks of infection in hospitals, the avoidance of trouble by pharmacies speaks volumes for the skill and discipline of pharmacists. The maintenance of this good record requires detailed agreement on policies between pharmacists and infection control staff, the results being incorporated into the Infection Control Manual.

Pharmacy design, like that of operating theatres, is a skilled business. Proper attention must be given to the segregation of 'clean' and 'dirty' areas. Production work must be organized on a basis of avoidance of contact between 'clean' and 'dirty' materials, with a proper flow of production work towards the autoclaves and safe storage of products thereafter. Filtered air must be passed by positive pressure ventilation from 'clean' to 'dirty' areas and not be allowed to recirculate. There must be adequate room for the storage and quarantine of stocks until quality control testing is complete. There must be careful attention to sterile water supply, drainage, and the washability of surfaces.

Cleaning schedules and protocols for environmental testing of sterile production areas should be agreed. The routine, planned, preventive maintenance of autoclaves and their in-use testing using thermocouples with chart recorders should be considered and agreed procedures should be enshrined in the Manual.

When possible, pharmacies should undertake any addition of drugs to intravenous fluids rather than this being undertaken by staff at the bedside. The procedures to be followed in an intravenous fluid additive service of this kind should be defined in writing.

The Control of Infection Committee should agree on a suitable range of disinfectants to be used for various purposes. This range of products, and no others, should be stocked by the pharmacy staff who effectively then police the disinfectant policy. Since most clinicians are not well informed about disinfectants, it is probable that such a disinfectant policy will raise the standard of disinfection by ensuring the use of appropriate substances only. A well constructed policy is also capable of saving a lot of money.

Antibiotic prescribing policies (see Chapter 4) may be in use, in which case the pharmacy may have another important part to play in providing advice. It will, in any case, be a major source of information on drug costs, and on prescribing patterns.

Central sterile supply

When the importance of using sterile surgical instruments was recognized in the nineteenth century, the only available means of sterilization was immersion in boiling water. This proved unsatisfactory because bacterial spores survived exposure to boiling water; because the penetration of boiling water into the interstices of instruments was not reliable; because it was not easy to ensure that instruments were left in the boiler for long enough, and because, after treatment, they were wet, thus facilitating transfer of organisms from the dresser's hands to the wound. Boiling waterbaths gave way to autoclaves, large containers in which instruments could be exposed to high temperature steam after the evacuation of air by the drawing of a vacuum. Autoclaves became more and more complicated, so requiring more skilled staff for their proper use, more careful quality control, and the expenditure of large sums of money for their purchase and maintenance. It gradually became apparent that the production of sterile equipment for hospital use would benefit from rationalization, and so central sterile supply departments were introduced. This centralization resulted in improvement in the standard of sterilizing, improved quality control, improved choice and maintenance of autoclaves, planned replacement of autoclaves, reduction in the number of autoclaves in use, and marked manpower savings.

As time went by, the work of these departments was concentrated on the production of sterile equipment and materials for use in the wards and outpatient departments, the preparation of packs of instruments and other items for use in operating theatres being undertaken in theatre sterile supply units. Sometimes these units were sited together, sometimes not. These arrangements did not cover the need for cleaning, overhauling, maintaining and disinfecting equipment which was in contact with patients, but which would not withstand heat sterilization. Such equipment may contain delicate electronic components, or be made of heat sensitive plastics, and includes baby incubators, ventilators, humidifiers, anaesthetic machines, heart—lung machines and endoscopes. Such apparatus may be processed in a medical equipment disinfection unit by exposure to warm water washing and thorough drying, to formaldehyde vapour, or to ethylene oxide gas.

Nowadays it is desirable that all hospital sterilizing activity should be concentrated in the three types of unit: the central and theatre sterile supply units and the medical equipment disinfection unit. It will often be sensible to organize these services in such a way that they serve not just one, but many hospitals. The organization of such services, and the procedures used, should be a concern of the Control of Infection Committee, and the procedures used should be described in the Infection Control Manual.

Some of the equipment in contact with patients cannot be properly sterilized without damage. A current problem is posed by fibre optic endoscopes which would be damaged by heat or formaldehyde vapour. Such endoscopes are usually disinfected by immersion in glutaraldehyde, a process which does not ensure sterilization. Equipment which cannot be sterilized should not be introduced into medical practice without good reason. Clinicians wishing to introduce new equipment should obtain clearance from the Control of Infection Committee who will advise on suitable decontamination procedures.

Operating theatres

The operating theatre is a prime location for the introduction of organisms to vulnerable sites, whether the organisms are derived from the patient's own flora or not. As has already been indicated, some of the risks can be minimized by theatre design, including provision of appropriate air flow by positive pressure ventilation. Suitably devised operational policies are also required, and these should be described in the Infection Control Manual. Thought should be given to protective clothing, masks, skin preparation, handwashing, and the like. Theatre cleaning schedules should be worked out. Special arrangements will be necessary for handling patients with particular infectious problems such as open pulmonary tuberculosis, or hepatitis. 'Dirty' cases, such as already infected wounds or acute peritonitis, should be handled in separate operating theatres from 'clean' cases. If that is not possible, 'dirty' cases should be dealt with at the end of an operating list, to minimize the chance of infecting clean wounds.

Kitchens

Hospital kitchens daily prepare vast numbers of meals for patients and staff. Large outbreaks of food poisoning or intestinal infection are therefore possible, and great care must be taken to avoid them. Washing facilities must be adequate, and the staff must be instructed in the importance of their use. Kitchen staff suffering from diarrhoea or vomiting should be taken off duty until cleared to return to work. Those developing infections on their hands should also be temporarily relieved of their duties.

Regular inspections of the kitchens should be undertaken to make sure that proper procedures are followed. The temperatures at which refrigerators and freezers work should be checked. Cooked and uncooked food should not come into contact with each other. Work surfaces should be clean and smooth. Slow cooling of cooked food should not be permitted. Kitchen utensils should be clean and dry. Waste should be promptly removed. Attention should be given to control of flies and cockroaches, and the kitchens should be kept free of mice, rats, cats and dogs.

The catering officer should be responsible for ensuring that the kitchens operate in a hygienic way, calling in colleagues for advice when necessary. He should be a member of the Control of Infection Committee. From time to time, the Public Health authorities should be invited to inspect the kitchens to advise on any hazards they may observe.

Pest control

In various parts of the hospital, sundry pests will constitute an infective risk because of the pathogenic organisms which they may carry. Regular checks should be made for signs of the presence of rats, mice, cats, pigeons, cockroaches, Pharaoh's ants, flies or other interlopers. In malarial areas, mosquito control may be a problem. Every member of staff should be asked to report 'sightings' of pests. No effort should be spared to control this type of nuisance. The responsibility for arranging for surveillance and control of pests should be vested in a suitable person who should report to the Control of Infection Committee.

Occupational health

Staff health departments in hospitals often undertake two kinds of work: (1) primary medical care of resident staff (a duplication of general practitioner services), and (2) health care of hospital workers regarding specific risks related to their employment. As far as infection control is concerned, both types of activity are relevant.

Members of staff who develop certain kinds of infection may represent a risk to patients or to other workers. Surgical staff with sore throats caused by haemolytic streptococci or with staphylococcal infections of the hands may give rise to infected surgical wounds. Nursing or medical staff with acute upper respiratory tract infections may transmit these to their patients. Catering staff with intestinal infections or staphylococcal hand infections may cause gastrointestinal infections or food poisoning in staff or patients. Staff with some infectious diseases such as rubella or chicken pox may infect patients in their care. Such examples indicate the need for staff health departments to agree policies with the Control of Infection Committee as to which unwell staff should be taken off duty.

Immunization policies for staff in contact with patients should be agreed. This will have benefits in protecting staff from acquiring some infections from patients, and *vice versa*. At University College Hospital, clinical staff are immunized against rubella (if not already immune), poliomyelitis and tetanus, and are offered BCG immunization against tuberculosis if Mantoux test negative. They are also offered a chest X-ray at suitable intervals if their work is likely to bring them into contact with tuberculous patients or material. Enough has already been said to indicate that different groups of hospital staff run different risks, and represent various degrees of threat to patients and other staff. Policies related to infection control must be designed to fit a realistic assessment of need.

'Sharps'

Apart from the various staff health matters already discussed, a variety of safe procedures for staff to use in hospitals must be devised. One recurrent problem is that of the safe disposal of sharp objects which may cause lacerations to those handling them. Examples of such 'sharps' include needles, intravenous drip sets, disposable scalpel blades and glass ampoules. Many of these will be contaminated with patients' blood and so represent a possible infective hazard as well as the risk of physical injury. Although several different infections could be transmitted by such inoculation injuries, the one which causes most anxiety is hepatitis B.

Carefully devised procedures for the safe disposal of 'sharps' must be introduced and the staff must be educated to implement them. If, despite this, a member of staff injures himself on a potentially infected 'sharp' he should be required to present himself at once in the staff health department. Inquiry should be made as to whether the source of the 'sharp' is known. If the patient on whom it was used is a carrier of the hepatitis B surface antigen (HBsAg), the injured staff member should be offered immune globulin at once, with a positive recommendation that it be accepted. If the patient is known not to be HBsAg positive, immune globulin should not be given. If the source of the 'sharp' is not known, the staff member should be offered immune globulin with advice as to the chance of the patient being HBsAg positive. The chance of this in the United Kingdom is about 0.1%, but it is higher in some other countries. Blood should be taken from any such injured employee when he is seen in the Staff Health Unit to establish that he was HBsAg negative at the time of injury. If he develops HBsAg positive hepatitis at the usual interval after injury, the employee will then be able to establish that this is an occupational disease entitling him to appropriate financial benefits.

Laboratory safety

Samples sent to the laboratories for pathological examination are commonly infected with micro-organisms, which potentially represent a risk to laboratory staff. This is true whether the specimens are sent to microbiology laboratories or to others (including post-mortem rooms). Laboratory workers have always been aware of the risks associated with handling infected materials and have, over the years, devised relatively safe working procedures. There is still, however, an excess incidence of hepatitis and tuberculosis in workers in clinical laboratories which has given rise to a demand for safer working conditions. In my own time in microbiology, I have seen two colleagues contract typhoid fever, one paratyphoid fever and one bacillary dysentery, all from clinical material.

There have been two outbreaks of smallpox derived from virus laboratories in the United Kingdom in recent years. These, and well publicized laboratory mishaps with Lassa fever virus and Ebola fever virus, have led to irresistible pressure from staff organizations to tighten up the controls on clinical laboratories. In the United Kingdom, this has resulted in the production of the Howie Report (1979) the recommendations in which, on the prevention of infection in clinical laboratories and post-mortem rooms, have been accepted by government. The Report requires large numbers of restrictive changes in work pattern which many British pathologists consider excessive, but which must, by law, be introduced. One reasonable requirement is that there must be a locally devised set of safe laboratory procedures for use in each department. These local arrangements should be notified to the Control of Infection Committee. It may be expected that similar controls on laboratory work will be introduced for similar reasons in other countries where they do not already exist. It is to be hoped that when this occurs it will be done without hampering laboratory work, and with less prodigal waste of money than has been the case in the United Kingdom.

Paediatrics

Paediatric wards present infectious hazards in at least two ways: because of the likelihood that children will be admitted suffering from the early (but infectious) stages of communicable diseases before these are easily recognized, and because small children are very mobile and play in close contact with each other in the ward. The source of infection is therefore constantly present, together with a ready means of transmission.

As far as possible, children with diarrhoea, prodromal measles, chicken pox and the like should not be admitted to general paediatric wards. In case of doubt, they should be barrier nursed to minimize spread of infection. A rapid diagnostic service should be made available in an attempt to avoid unnecessary restrictions on the management of sick children in the wards. Children found to have highly transmissible respiratory pathogens should be transferred to an infectious diseases unit.

The neonatal intensive care unit presents special problems because numbers of very frail, ill babies are gathered together in one place and because these babies need intravenous catheters, ventilators and humidifiers for life support. Overwhelming infection of these very small babies, caused by Gram-negative bacilli or by Group B haemolytic streptococci, is common. Screening procedures for *Pseudomonas aeruginosa* and haemolytic streptococci in neonates admitted to the unit and at weekly intervals thereafter may be helpful.

Intravenous catheter tips and intravenous fluid filters should be cultured for bacteria routinely. A policy should be agreed for the microbiological investigation of babies whose clinical state is deteriorating.

Detailed care should be taken in devising nursing procedures; in the provision and use of protective clothing, gloves and masks; in the decontamination and sterilization of equipment, and in the provision and use of isolation facilities. All this should be kept under review by the Control of Infection Committee. Clinical microbiologists should visit neonatal units daily, not only to attend to sick babies, but also to watch how infection control procedures are working out in practice.

Intensive care units

The problems here are very like those in neonatal units, and the Control of Infection Committee and the microbiologists should be taking an interest in the same way. In both types of unit, it may be necessary to limit the use of certain antibiotics (Chapter 4) in an attempt to prevent colonization of patients by, and subsequent infection with, certain antibiotic-resistant Gram-negative organisms. This type of policy depends upon the willingness and ability of clinical microbiologists to visit the unit at least once daily and to advise on antibiotic choice. Such visits provide an opportunity to observe how medical and nursing procedures are carried out and to suggest possible improvements calculated to reduce the risks of infection.

Haemodialysis

Units performing dialysis, whether haemodialysis or peritoneal dialysis, expose patients, and perhaps staff, to special risks. There is the utmost need for scrupulous hygiene in this environment, for careful cleaning and disinfection of equipment, and for meticulous attention to detailed working procedures by clinical staff. A particular problem with haemodialysis in the past has been the risk of outbreaks of hepatitis B in patients and staff. Transfusion blood is now screened to exclude donations from people carrying the viral antigen (HBsAg), so greatly reducing the risk. Haemodialysis units should routinely screen staff and patients on admission, to ensure that they are HBsAg negative. Patients found to be antigen positive should be isolated and dialysed outside the unit by staff especially instructed in the procedures to be used. If possible, such patients should be dialysed in their own homes using their own equipment. Results of improved methods have been satisfactory, so that the risks are now slight.

Burns units

The risk of infection of extensive burns is obvious. Infection may be endogenous or exogenous. Exogenous infection may be airborne, or transmitted on the hands of attending staff. Patients with extensive burns should be barrier nursed in separate rooms. Dressings should be changed in an operating theatre when possible, using full aseptic precautions. Whenever possible the use of broad spectrum antibiotics should be avoided, and antimicrobial prophylaxis should be eschewed. The Control of Infection Committee should take an active interest in the procedures used in burns units, and the clinical microbiologists should visit regularly.

Surveillance

None of the problems mentioned above are capable of satisfactory resolution without constant attention from all interested parties. Infections are not prevented without considerable effort. The Control of Infection Committee must be a strongly led force for change, but it must have good and demonstrable reasons for its recommendations.

In order that the Committee can perform its duties effectively, its advice must be sought on relevant matters, and its recommendations must be implemented. The Committee must ensure that appropriate issues are brought to it and debated fully, and that its advice is constructive and capable of implementation.

It is all too easy for people to sit around a committee table, thinking up ways in which infections might occur and devising means of preventing each one. They leave feeling satisfied that no stone has been left unturned. However, senior staff members may have lost touch to some extent with day to day realities of the work which may have changed since they were doing it. The outcome is often recommendations which may be unnecessarily complex and time consuming so that, in practice, they are not carried out. The advice of the infection control committee will then not be taken seriously and confidence in its work will be lost. When introducing a new anti-infection measure, the committee must be sure that, as individuals, they would insist on it being carried out whatever shortage of staff or other difficult circumstances may arise. If it is not as important as that, its value is dubious. A major problem for such committees is to ensure that there is a good system of infection reporting, so that members can bring their attention to bear on current problems. Much will depend on the existence of harmonious relationships between microbiologists, and the infection control nurses and other nursing and medical staff from whom they receive information.

The implementation of existing policies, and the introduction of new ones alike, depend on a programme of continuing education of all health workers, whether trainees or permanent staff. Ensuring that this is satisfactorily undertaken is a major function of Control of Infection Committees. Whenever an outbreak is brought under control, its features should be analysed and any lessons learned brought to the attention of all concerned. In this way all can learn how to improve future infection control.

9

The control of
antibiotic resistance

No man is an Island, entire of it self.
Any man's death diminishes me, because I am involved in Mankind;
And therefore never send to know for whom the bell tolls; It tolls for thee.

Devotions, John Donne (1571?—1631)

Each generation of medical microbiologists faces new clinical challenges, as indicated in Chapter 7. A major preoccupation at present is the spread of antibiotic resistant bacteria which threaten the effectiveness of antimicrobial chemotherapy. This is an ever increasing problem which is beginning to pose new problems in clinical management.

Antibiotic resistance existed in bacteria before the introduction of antimicrobial agents. Changes in bacterial susceptibility to antibiotics have been brought about by mutation, adaptation, conjugation, transduction and transformation (see Chapter 4). The use of antibiotics has acted as a potent selective pressure, promoting the accumulation of resistant bacteria, as sensitive organisms are eliminated. The present high degree of antibiotic resistance in the bacterial flora is undoubtedly a result of the increasing worldwide use of antimicrobial drugs.

The international nature of this phenomenon is noteworthy. Even in communities in those remote areas of Papua New Guinea in which antibiotics have scarcely been used, it has been found that antibiotic

151

resistant bacteria are isolated from infected lesions and from the faecal flora of healthy people. The human bacterial flora should be regarded as one ecological entity, with organisms moving freely about the world without regard to political frontiers. Newly antibiotic-resistant strains of bacteria spread from country to country, carrying their resistances with them. Examples in recent years include the spread of chloramphenicol-resistant *Salmonella typhi* from Mexico, of penicillin-resistant *Neisseria gonorrhoeae* from the Philippines, of sulphonamide-resistant *N. meningitidis* from the U.S.A., and of penicillin-resistant pneumococci from S. Africa. It follows that the problems of antibiotic resistance in medically important bacteria are global, requiring an international approach.

In Chapter 4, I discussed an approach to antibiotic prescribing policies in hospitals. Such policies are generally introduced when antibiotic treatment in a hospital unit is becoming seriously circumscribed because of accumulating resistances in pathogenic bacteria. The general argument is that the more an antibiotic is used, the greater the prevalence of bacteria resistant to it: withdraw the antibiotic and the bacteria may be expected to revert to antibiotic sensitivity. The literature is full of accounts of outbreaks of antibiotic-resistant infections controlled in just this way. Sometimes, however, the problem is more involved, and requires more careful analysis for its resolution.

An outbreak of hospital infection

By way of an example of a complex situation, I propose to describe a hospital outbreak of trimethoprim resistance in pathogenic coliform bacilli which was reported from one of the hospitals in the University College Hospital Group (Grüneberg and Bendall, 1979).

In 1971, we showed that some patients in St. Pancras Hospital had infections caused by coliform bacilli carrying R-factors mediating trimethoprim (TMP) resistance, and that similar organisms could be found in the bowel flora of the infected patients and of some others. In the summer of 1971, we realized that many coliform pathogens from patients in St. Pancras Hospital were TMP-resistant. Many of the infections were of the urinary tract, and most occurred in the geriatric wards. Whereas most of the earlier TMP-resistant organisms were *Escherichia coli*, gradually *Klebsiella* spp. became predominant.

Because of the recognition of a link between infection and carriage in the bowel, the outbreak was investigated by screening the whole inpatient population of the hospital for rectal carriage of TMP-resistant, coliform bacilli. Table 7 shows the results of that screening (July–August 1972). Of the 278 patients screened, 49 (17.6%) were found to be carriers, and of these, 41 were in the four geriatric wards.

Table 7   Results of screening inpatients for rectal carriage of TMP-resistant coliform bacilli

Ward	Type	July-Aug 1972	Mar 1973	Apr 1973	July 1973	Jan 1974	Aug 1974	Sep 1975	Oct 1976
		No. of carriers/no. of patients screened							
1	Female surgical	0/18		0/13	1/24	0/5	1/9	0/10	
3	Male surgical	1/22		2/16	1/16	0/6	2/15	2/16	
4	Male medical	1/20		2/15	2/20	7/20	3/23	1/14	
5	Male geriatric	13/26	5/22	6/26	5/24	5/25	7/17	2/24†	0/19
6	Female medical	3/24		6/25	2/20	0/22	0/19	2/16	
7	Female geriatric	15/29	4/29	2/30*	2/28	2/22	0/23	3/23	1/16
8	Female geriatric	11/26	2/27	2/29	2/26	6/26	12/27	1/23†	1/19
9	Mixed geriatric	2/21	4/19	2/19	Closed	6/22	6/25	2/19†	1/21
NWM	Male psychiatric	0/20		0/26	0/24	0/16	0/13	0/16	
NWF	Female psychiatric	0/25		0/21	0/19	1/23	0/15	0/17	
Manson	Mixed tropical	2/25		0/24	1/18	0/19	0/12	0/24	
Chamberlain	Mixed tropical	1/22		0/13	0/20	0/20	1/20	0/25	
Total		49/278		22/257	16/239	27/226	32/218	13/227	
Wards 5,7,8,9 (all geriatric)		41/102	15/97	12/104		19/95	25/92	8/89	3/75

*No sulphonamide, ampicillin, or co-trimoxazole used in ward 7 from 1 April 1973
†No sulphonamide, ampicillin, or co-trimoxazole used in wards 5, 8 and 9 from 1 December 1974

Investigation of the carrier state
We confined the analysis to the occupants of the four geriatric wards (wards 5, 7, 8 and 9) and examined the case notes of 100 of the 102 patients concerned.

Influence of sex of patient

The carrier rate among the men (50%) was not much different from that among the women (47.3%).

Table 8 Average ages (±SD) of geriatric patients in relation to carrier state

	Carriers		Non-carriers		p value for difference
	No.	Age (years)	No.	Age (years)	
Men	13	79.3 ± 9.4	14	73.6 ± 7.5	≤ 0.001
Women	28	84.6 ± 8.0	45	79.8 ± 7.7	≤ 0.001

Influence of age of patient

Significant differences in carrier rate with age were found, older patients of either sex being more likely to be carriers ($p \leqslant 0.001$), as shown in Table 8.

Table 9 Relationship between timing of latest treatment with any antimicrobial agent and carrier state

Interval before screening (months)	Carriers (n = 41)		Non-carriers (n = 59)		Significance of difference $[\chi^2]$
	No. (%) treated	No. not treated	No. (%) treated	No. not treated	
0—1	15(36.6)	26	8(13.6)	51	$p \leqslant 0.01$
0—3	23(56.1)	18	15(25.4)	44	$p \leqslant 0.01$
0—6	31(75.6)	10	24(40.7)	35	$p \leqslant 0.01$
0—12	34(82.9)	7	27(45.8)	32	$p \leqslant 0.01$
0—12+	35(85.4)	6	39(66.1)	20	$p \leqslant 0.01$

Table 10 Number of courses of chemotherapy before screening in relation to carrier state

Interval before screening (months)	Carriers (n = 41)		Non-carriers (n = 59)	
	Total no. of courses	Average no./ patient	Total no. of courses	Average no./ patient
0—1	20	0.5	10	0.2
0—3	37	0.9	23	0.4
0—6	73	1.8	39	0.7
0—12	100	2.4	57	1.0
0—12+	129	3.1	85	1.4

Table 11   Relationship between timing of latest treatment with co-trimoxazole, sulphonamides, or ampicillin and carrier state

Interval before screening (months)	Carriers (n = 41)		Non-carriers (n = 59)		Significance of difference [χ^2]
	No. (%) treated	No. not treated	No. (%) treated	No. not treated	
0–1	15(36.6)	28	4(6.6)	55	$p \leqslant 0.01$
0–3	21(51.2)	20	9(15.2)	50	$p \leqslant 0.01$
0–6	27(65.9)	14	17(28.8)	42	$p \leqslant 0.01$
0–12	30(73.2)	11	19(32.2)	40	$p \leqslant 0.01$
0–12+	30(73.2)	11	21(35.6)	38	$p \leqslant 0.01$

Table 12   Number of courses of co-trimoxazole, sulphonamides, or ampicillin before screening in relation to carrier state

Interval before screening (months)	Carriers (n = 41)		Non-carriers (n = 59)	
	Total no. of courses	Average no./ patient	Total no. of courses	Average no./ patient
0–1	16	0.4	6	0.1
0–3	32	0.8	18	0.3
0–6	63	1.5	33	0.6
0–12	88	2.1	44	0.7
0–12+	144	2.8	68	1.2

Influence of exposure to antimicrobial agents before screening

Table 9 shows that patients were more likely to be carriers ($p \leqslant 0.01$) if they had previously been given an antimicrobial agent. Carriers were about twice as likely as non-carriers to have received chemotherapy within about six months before screening. That carriers were more likely to have had chemotherapy than non-carriers is also shown in Table 10 as is the fact that carriers were also likely to have had more courses of antimicrobials than non-carriers. Tables 11 and 12 show that the important drugs were co-trimoxazole, sulphonamides, and ampicillin. Analysis showed that, in both sexes, those patients above the group mean ages (76.3 years for men and 81.6 years for women) were significantly more likely ($p \leqslant 0.05$) to have received some chemo-

therapy, or to have received treatment with co-trimoxazole, sulphonamides, or ampicillin, within the previous three months than patients
below the group mean age. The size of this effect was such as to
establish that the fact that older people were more likely to be carriers
(Table 8) was almost, but not entirely, explicable on the basis of
greater antibiotic exposure.

Influence of duration of hospital stay before screening

The average duration of stay in hospital before screening of geriatric
patients was 14.9 months in carriers and 8.1 months in non-carriers. A
detailed factorial analysis showed that older patients of either sex
stayed in hospital longer, received more antimicrobial chemotherapy
(and more treatment with co-trimoxazole, sulphonamides, or ampicillin), and were more likely to become carriers of TMP-resistant coliform bacilli than younger patients. By far the most important of these
factors was treatment with co-trimoxazole, sulphonamides, or ampicillin in the previous months, but duration of hospital stay also contributed.

*Summary of analysis of factors determining likelihood of developing
carrier state*

The main predisposing factor to rectal carriage of TMP-resistant
organisms was previous antimicrobial chemotherapy, particularly
with co-trimoxazole, sulphonamides, or ampicillin. The age of the
patient, and the duration of stay in hospital before screening, predisposed mainly in so far as they affected exposure to chemotherapy,
although duration of stay in hospital also predisposed independently.
Presumably, the longer a patient stayed in hospital the more likely he
was to be in contact with a carrier and the longer such contact would
be maintained, so that his own chances of becoming a carrier were
increased. The sex of the patient was not a predisposing factor,
probably because the exposure to antibiotics was similar for both
sexes.

Attempts at solution

By the time this analysis was completed, we had satisfied ourselves that the carrier state was of practical importance. Between July 1972 and February 1974 some 105 patients were found to be carriers. Of these, 38 (36.2%) developed clinical infections recognized as being caused by TMP-resistant coliform organisms, but this is certainly an underestimate of the actual number of such infections occurring. While most TMP-resistant infections were minor, all degrees of severity were seen, including two cases of septicaemia, one of which was fatal. The rectal flora of patients who developed infections with TMP-resistant coliforms yielded similar organisms in 88% of cases.

We chose two similar geriatric wards (7 and 8) for further study. Each housed about 30 patients on the same landing of the hospital. They had common medical but separate nursing staff. It was agreed that in ward 7, co-trimoxazole, sulphonamides, and ampicillin would not be used from 1 April 1973, while in ward 8, the medical staff would use whatever chemotherapy was thought appropriate. Any patients in ward 7 needing a restricted drug would be transferred elsewhere (this happened only once). Table 7 shows the results of screening just before the beginning of the experiment (March 1973) and again in April 1973, January 1974, and August 1974. The level of TMP-resistant carriage was similar in wards 7 and 8 at the beginning of this period. After nine months (January 1974), two out of 22 patients in ward 7 and six out of 26 patients in ward 8 were carriers. After 15 months (August 1974) no carriers were detected among 23 patients in ward 7, whereas in ward 8, 12 out of 27 patients were carriers. In parallel with this clearance of TMP-resistant coliforms from the rectal flora of patients in ward 7, no episodes of urinary tract infection caused by such organisms occurred between May 1973 and August 1974 in that ward. In contrast, in ward 8, where carriage of TMP-resistant coliforms continued, nine urinary tract infections due to these organisms occurred during the same period.

From 1 December 1974, the antibiotic restrictions in force in ward 7 were extended to all four geriatric wards (5, 7, 8 and 9). By October 1976, only three carriers remained among the 75 patients in the four wards (Table 7). TMP-resistant coliforms as a cause of infection had virtually disappeared. Thus, newly introduced policies restricting antibiotics produced their maximum effect in about nine months. Of 326 resistant strains of *Escherichia coli* and *Klebsiella* spp. isolated from infections or from rectal flora between 1970 and the summer of 1973, 278 had an MIC (minimum inhibitory concentration) of TMP of $\geqslant 1000\,\mu g/ml$. Thus 85% of the TMP-resistant coliform organisms isolated had the extremely high MIC associated with plasmid mediated TMP resistance. Among the TMP-resistant *E. coli* isolated from various sources in the hospital during this outbreak 16 different O-serotypes were identified.

When an outbreak of this sort occurs, careful analysis may give the key to effective remedial action. This is probably best undertaken jointly by clinicians and laboratory staff. Without such collaboration in this case, the crucial importance of exposure of patients to ampicillin might have been missed. The point was that the organisms carrying the W plasmid mediating TMP resistance were mostly *E. coli* strains at the beginning of the outbreak, but gradually strains of *Klebsiella* spp. became predominant. Since the klebsiellae are inherently resistant to ampicillin, use of the drug will select these organisms, TMP plasmid included. Thus, using an apparently irrelevant antibiotic may select for unrelated resistances. Once the team has established the relevant facts, resolute and logically selected policies, jointly implemented, may be expected to control the outbreak, as in this case.

'Wider yet, and wider . . .'

In this episode, it was necessary to control the use not only of apparently relevant drugs, but also of an apparently irrelevant one before the problem of antibiotic resistance receded. Although the problem of trimethoprim-resistant coliform infection began in geriatric wards, it spread to other wards within the hospital. Cases occurred in other hospitals in the group, and among patients attending general practitioners in the neighbourhood. Although it may be usual in medicine to think in compartmentalized terms, bacteria and their resistances do not behave in that way. Under normal circumstances, there will be a slow movement of micro-organisms from person to person in a community, supplemented perhaps by widescale dissemination of organisms in food or drink. This slow rate of change will ensure that the microbes found in one locality are slightly different from those in another neighbourhood nearby, and much different from those found at a great distance. An example of this was shown (Grüneberg and Bettelheim, 1969) in strains of *Escherichia coli* isolated from urinary tract infections in general practice. The O-serotypes of *E. coli* reported from America and from Europe showed widely different distributions, and differences in prevalence could be shown in infections occurring in communities only a few kilometres apart. Similar findings could probably be shown for the antibiotic sensitivities of common organisms derived from different areas. Superimposed on this slow exchange of bacteria by personal contact, is the dramatic mobility of bacteria facilitated by the movement of their human hosts by air, or of human foodstuffs by sea. Bacteria have acquired a new propensity for rapid geographical spread occasioned by these changes in methods of human transport. With these bacteria will travel their antibiotic resistances.

The limitations of locally implemented antibiotic prescribing policies designed to minimize antibiotic resistance in pathogenic bacteria must now be obvious. Although a particular hospital's policy may be well devised and rigorously enforced, it will be at least partially negated by the lack of similar policies in other hospitals in the vicinity, and by the absence of any attempt at regulation of antibiotic use in general practice. Even if full agreement could be reached in a country on a suitable antibiotic prescribing policy for national use, and if it was implemented effectively, it would still not work completely, because resistant organisms would continually be invading from other, less controlled countries (a form of unrecognized 'germ warfare' unknowingly carried on by friendly states). So far only Czechoslovakia has seriously attempted to implement a policy of antibiotic restraint (Modr, 1978). What would make much more sense, if mankind were only organized politically in such a way as to facilitate it, would be a worldwide international agreement on antibiotic use designed to prevent the spread of antibiotic resistant bacteria. Any such international policy would have to be capable of rapid revision in the light of observed changes in the prevalence of antibiotic resistances. Patterns of bacterial antibiotic resistance would have to be monitored in many places around the world, and the results communicated to some centre for evaluation before the policy could be appropriately modified. Such a system might perhaps be introduced under the auspices of the World Health Organization.

The difficulties in making such arrangements would be formidable. In some countries antibiotics are only available on prescription, while in others they may be bought freely by the public. Many countries cannot afford to use the more expensive drugs which may sometimes be ecologically preferable to cheaper agents. Black market trafficking in antibiotics is common in some parts of the world. Such problems could be overcome, given the political will to do so, but it would not be easy.

Animal husbandry

With the best will in the world, there would remain another problem, in that antibiotics are not used only in human medicine. They are also used in the treatment of infected animals, and as a supplement to animal feedstuffs to make livestock gain weight more rapidly (by mechanisms that are not properly understood). Veterinarians are, no doubt, as concerned as medical practitioners to provide the best possible treatment for their patients, and their professional ethics might cause them to reject a proposition that some antibiotics should not be given to sick animals lest the value of those drugs to man be diminished. They might (with justice) point out that the diminished usefulness of tetracyclines in human infection has been caused by the use of those drugs in medical practice (Richmond and Linton, 1980) rather than in other applications. Accepting the need for the medical profession to put its own house in order, there must still be scope for the two professions to agree on policies acceptable to both.

A much more difficult problem is posed by the use of antibiotics in animal feedstuffs to enhance the rate of weight gain by domestic livestock. The commercial advantage of this practice is very great, so that it is not reasonable to expect it to be forgone by farmers. It is not unreasonable to expect, however, that those antibiotics used in human medicine should not be used as feed additives. The risk is that animal pathogens such as *Salmonella* spp. continuously exposed, for instance, to chloramphenicol will become resistant to that drug. If such organisms subsequently cause human infection, the usefulness of antibiotics will be reduced. Alternatively, the acquired resistances of such animal bacterial strains may be transferred to other intestinal organisms such as *Escherichia coli* or *Salmonella typhi*, more likely in due course to give rise to human invasive disease. The real fear is that *S. typhi* strains will become resistant to chloramphenicol, ampicillin/amoxycillin and trimethoprim, so leaving us without effective drugs against typhoid fever, a disease which, when left untreated, has a 5—15% mortality rate. The problem is made much more difficult by the fact, as demonstrated in the hospital outbreak described earlier in this chapter, that it is possible for the use of other drugs to select for the relevant resistances. Thus, it would be appropriate to use as animal feed additives only those drugs which are not used in human medicine, and bacterial resistance to which is not linked to resistances to medically important antibiotics. This would drastically reduce the number of drugs available for use in this way.

An attempt to control this application of antibiotics by law was made in the United Kingdom as a result of recommendations in the Swann Report (1969). The anxiety which led to the setting up of the Swann committee and to the enacting of legislation, was occasioned by the rapid spread and prevalence of antibiotic-resistant strains of *Salmonella typhimurium* from human and animal sources in the United Kingdom during the nineteen sixties, and the linking of these findings with the uncontrolled use of relevant antibiotics to supplement animal feedstuffs. The legislation divided antibiotics into two classes, those which were used for treatment of sick animals, and those which were used as feed additives. The latter had little or no therapeutic use and were made available without prescription. The therapeutic antimicrobial agents could be obtained for animal use only on prescription by a veterinary practitioner. Unfortunately, these regulations have not been as effective as was hoped, partly because of the existence of a black market in 'controlled' antibiotics, and partly because of the irresponsible use of therapeutic drugs by those who should know better. It has now become apparent (Threlfall *et al.*, 1980), due to the isolation from cattle and man of epidemic strains of *S. typhimurium* which have become resistant to ampicillin, chloramphenicol, kanamycin, streptomycin, sulphonamide, tetracycline and trimethoprim as a result of the prophylactic use in cattle of trimethoprim, that the Swann legislation has failed. Since man's health is directly threatened by such developments, it is vitally important that the regulations be tightened to make them more effective. New regulations must govern both veterinary and agricultural use of antibiotics.

The challenge

The stakes being played for are very high. Since the introduction of antimicrobial drugs fifty years ago, their use has transformed medical practice and the quality of human life. The limiting factor in the usefulness of antimicrobial drugs has been the prevalence of bacterial drug resistance. One drug after another has been reduced in its application by increasing bacterial resistance. So far, the pharmaceutical industry has managed to produce new antibiotics at a rate sufficient to match the loss of earlier drugs occasioned by bacterial changes. However, there is a considerable likelihood that new groups of antibiotics, strikingly different from those already available, will no longer flow from the pharmaceutical industry, new products being only marginal improvements on existing drugs. If that is so, the existing anarchic state of antibiotic use can be expected, in a few years, to lead to a changed bacterial environment in which antimicrobial chemotherapy will be ineffective. Should that happen, the passing of the 'Antibiotic Era' will be remembered as another great historical tragedy (like the Fall of the Roman Empire) contributed to, if not caused, by the folly of man.

It can be seen that man may be entering the last round of a very significant bout with the medically important bacteria. As indicated in the early chapters of this book, the bacteria have considerable advantages in this struggle as their vast populations and their short generation time give them enormous numbers of opportunities for rapid change when faced with an evolutionary challenge such as the appearance of new antibiotics. There is, however, some evidence suggesting that bacteria which acquire antibiotic resistances are at a disadvantage, compared with sensitive strains, in the absence of antimicrobial agents. This means that if antibiotics are not used, the bacterial population gradually reverts to drug sensitivity. The lesson is clear: antibiotic use must be reduced to the minimum required to treat serious infection.

Man is not helpless when faced with this situation. He has enormous capacity to respond to a challenge, a soaring intellect, ability to communicate around the globe and the potential to organize himself. What is needed is much more awareness of the nature of the problem, and the generation of the political will to act decisively. The attitude of the medical profession, and of medical microbiologists in particular, will be of great importance in this. Bacterial resistance to antibiotics is a worldwide public health problem, and should be treated as such. It is more complicated than the eradication of smallpox and will require the application of far more resources, but at least partial success is attainable.

On a more personal scale, each doctor should make a start by reviewing his own antibiotic prescribing methods (see Chapter 4), and by pressing for the implementation of sensible antibiotic prescribing policies for use in his area. In hospitals, the development of such policies is still more important. Even with such policies in use, there will, for the foreseeable future, be sporadic outbreaks of infections caused by antibiotic resistant bacteria, such as that described earlier in this chapter. These will require careful evaluation and thoughtfully considered corrective action for their control. As suggested in Chapter 8, hospital infection and its control is moving into a new phase, that of the control of antibiotic resistance.

10

Medical microbiology in the future

> Of old when folk lay sick and sorely tried
> The doctors gave them physic, and they died.
> But here's a happier age: for now we know
> Both how to make men sick and keep them so.
>
> *On Hygiene*, Hilaire Belloc (1870—1953)

Men and microbes coexist in a very complicated relationship, such that the presence and activities of each profoundly affects the other in dozens of different ways. In order to consider how the future of this 'special relationship' may change, I shall assume that man does not destroy his settled communities by war, and that the current levels of overall material prosperity are maintained.

It may be expected that for several decades to come there will be a continuing increase in human population. I have seen projections suggesting a world population of about 15,000 million people by the middle of the next century. If this happens, it will be partly because infant mortality continues to fall, and partly because more adults survive into old age. Such population growth will probably not be evenly distributed but will affect poorer societies more profoundly than those which are relatively affluent. The growth of cities in the less prosperous countries will probably continue. These developments will pose enormous problems of social organization. Even with a benevolent, highly efficient world government single-mindedly dedicated to universal human welfare, it seems unlikely that such numbers could be fed, clothed and housed properly, and that cities could be provided with clean water supplies or adequate sewage disposal on the necessary scale. It seems probable to me that utopian government of this sort will not be achieved, and that the plight of vast numbers of people will worsen rather than improve. This will probably mean that many of the great infective scourges of mankind will remain prevalent and may, indeed, contribute to the limitation of human populations at a new, higher level. If the efforts of governments in many less prosperous countries become more effective in limiting population growth than they have been so far, populations may stabilize at a less high level with consequent improvement in the prevailing conditions. This would mean much less likelihood of famine and pestilence.

As long as no very striking improvement in the control of contagious diseases in the so-called third world occurs, it will never be possible in more prosperous communities to stamp out diseases such as tuberculosis completely. Increased freedom of travel (not to mention forced migrations) will lead to a continuing flow of the well recognized infections from the poorer communities in which they are common to their more fortunate neighbours. Additionally, it is to be expected that more patients incubating less well recognized infections will arrive in societies not expecting them, so repeating the experiences we have had with Lassa fever, Ebola fever and Marburg disease over the last decade or two. Such diseases are unlikely to establish themselves in a new environment because of lack of animal reservoirs or insect vectors, but their occasional arrival and the possibility of outcrops of secondary infections will, no doubt, give rise to public anxiety.

As described in Chapter 7, a wide range of immunizations is available against a variety of infectious agents. In recent years there has been a renewal of research interest in immunization. This has partly been concerned with the development of vaccines which are more specific, more effective and less likely to produce unwanted effects, and partly been directed at the production of vaccines protecting against infections for which protection has not previously been available.

We now have vaccines against rabies which can be more easily administered and are less likely to produce side effects; more specific vaccines against whooping cough; vaccines against enteric fever which can be given in low dosage intradermally, so avoiding many of the systemic side effects of the older vaccines; and much more strain-specific influenza vaccines. This process of refinement of existing immunizations can confidently be expected to continue in years to come. It is at present fashionable to decry the achievements of 'high technology' acute medical care, and to urge that resources be transferred from that field to the area of preventive medicine where money can be much more effectively spent. Although the validity of that argument is almost entirely unproved, one sphere in which it is certainly correct is that of immunization against infection. (It is interesting, though, that the development of vaccines is nowadays a very advanced technology, depending on tissue culture, viral recombination and 'genetic engineering'.) No doubt much more effort will in future be made to ensure a high uptake of available immunizations.

New vaccines are being developed apace. Work is proceeding on the prevention of cytomegalovirus (CMV) infection. Research on the production of vaccines preventing hepatitis A and hepatitis B is going forward rapidly. The use of vaccines to prevent *Pseudomonas aeruginosa* infections occurring in compromised patients in hospital is a very real possibility.

Sometimes, familiar infections change their characteristics or their geographical range. One example of this has been the replacement of the classical asiatic cholera by the el Tor vibrio and the successful establishment of the latter in Africa south of the Sahara desert. Another example has been the rapidly increasing prevalence of *Salmonella hadar* (derived from turkeys) in human intestinal infections in the UK in the last decade. The causes of such changes are not usually known, and it seems probable that more will occur in the years to come.

In recent years, the pathogenic importance of a number of organisms in human infection has been newly recognized (e.g. *Legionella pneumophila* as a cause of pneumonia, *Campylobacter* spp. causing intestinal infection, and *Chlamydia trachomatis* causing some cases of non-gonococcal urethritis, neonatal pneumonia and pelvic inflammatory disease). The increasing importance of micrococci as a cause of urinary tract infection in sexually active young women is another example. Some of these 'new' pathogens may arise because of changes in human activity (greater use of air-conditioning, intensive farming of livestock, changes in sexual custom) while others reflect the use of different laboratory procedures leading to recognition of previously unsuspected pathogenetic relationships. Research work is constantly refining our knowledge in this area, and no doubt further pathogens will be identified as causes of existing infections in the future.

Increasingly, it is being recognized that there may be an infective component in the causation of many diseases not traditionally thought to have one. Many workers have sought, so far unsuccessfully, infective causes for such diverse conditions as rheumatoid arthritis, regional ileitis (Crohn's disease) and ulcerative colitis. The pathological similarities between Creutzfeldt—Jakob disease and Kuru, both human diseases, and some degenerative neurological diseases in animals caused by 'slow viruses' have led to a search for similar viruses in man. Multiple sclerosis in man has pathological features in common with the viral diseases louping ill and scrapie in sheep, leading to a search for viruses which might be implicated in the human disease. I expect some such links to be established in the next few years.

Some cancers in experimental animals have, for very many years, been known to have viral causes. Despite enormous effort, it has not so far been possible to demonstrate that viruses are carcinogenic in man, although it seems very likely that they are. The closest approach to success here has been in the case of the maxillary tumour of the young, called Burkitt's lymphoma, which seems to be linked with a herpesvirus known as the Epstein—Barr virus. Human leukaemias seem so similar to animal leukaemias known to be caused by viruses that it is difficult to believe that viruses are not somehow implicated in them too.

Sometimes the suggested links between micro-organisms and disease are complicated. It has been suggested, for example, with supporting evidence, that different human dietary customs, such as eating a diet largely composed of plantains rather than a mixed diet, lead to quite different mixtures of aerobic and anaerobic bowel flora. Populations eating a mixed diet thus have an intestinal flora more capable of splitting bile salts into substances similar to known chemical carcinogens. Populations eating a mixed diet also have far more colonic cancers than do those eating the plantain diet (matoke) common in East Africa (Hill et al., 1971).

Research is proceeding on the involvement of micro-organisms in the causation of human tumours, and I expect to hear in years to come of the success of such work. Capitalizing on the results of such research by attempting to prevent cancers may still prove to be difficult, however, even if the causes of some tumours are recognized.

When I began my career in microbiology in the early nineteen sixties, clinical laboratories were very different from those of today. They were small and numerous, each employing few staff and receiving relatively few specimens. Culture media and laboratory reagents were home made and only a modest amount of equipment was in use, most of it cheap and locally produced. The work was undertaken using exclusively manual techniques. Morphological and cultural methods were relied heavily upon for bacterial identification, and were supplemented by simple chemical and serological tests. Clinical virology was in its infancy. We worked in cramped and, by present standards, dangerous laboratories. A large part of the available space was necessarily given over to media production, to washing up glassware, and to waste disposal. The prevailing approach to bacteriological work was morphological rather than functional, and qualitative rather than quantitative. The medical microbiologist was concerned only with laboratory diagnosis, and most stayed in their laboratories throughout their working day.

The change in the last two decades has been very profound and quite exciting. There are now far fewer clinical microbiology laboratories in the U.K. and those surviving are larger and undertake much more work. Several studies have shown that clinical laboratories have maintained a 10—14% per annum compound growth in workload for three decades. This greater level of work has forced massive changes in work pattern. Laboratory glassware has given way substantially to disposable plastics, reducing the need for glass washing, but posing new problems of waste disposal. An industry has grown up to supply ready made bacterial culture media, reducing the need for laboratories to prepare their own. Another industry has arisen to supply laboratory equipment on a vast scale, mostly of much improved design. The setting up of anaerobic cultures and the addition of carbon dioxide to improve growth have consequently become routine everywhere. New equipment dependent techniques are widespread, with the result that procedures which were very difficult to carry out manually are now easily performed in large numbers. Rapid techniques are available where previously they did not exist. The whole pace of laboratory activity has speeded up, and the administration of laboratories has grown in scale from that appropriate to a cottage industry, to that of a modern factory. Bigger laboratories are now using computers to handle data and to generate reports, and more importantly, to produce infection control information for hospital use.

The laboratory techniques in use now are much less concerned with bacterial morphology and much more concerned with the biochemical properties of bacteria than before. Chromatography, gas—liquid chromatography, antigen detection, antibody analysis by protein separation, electron microscopy and ultracentrifugation are the order of the day. Antibiotic sensitivity testing has made great strides in recent years, using mechanization and quantitative techniques. Bacterial counting is a routine activity. For technical reasons, mechanization has not moved as far or as fast in microbiology as in haematology and clinical chemistry, but the changes have, nonetheless, been remarkable. Quality control schemes are in widespread use so that laboratories can monitor their performance in various aspects of their clinical work. These are raising standards of practice, so that the gap in performance between the best laboratories and the average has narrowed.

I confidently expect the rapid rate of change in clinical microbiology laboratories to be maintained in the future. There will be further centralization of laboratories forced by the need to raise professional standards, by the need to achieve some economies of scale, by the need to meet stringent requirements in the field of laboratory safety, and because of difficulties in recruiting skilled staff. Such laboratory centralization has considerable benefits but it has the disadvantage of making the laboratories more remote from the patients and doctors they serve. It seems likely that the increase in workload of laboratories still has some way to run. This greater throughput of work will increase the pressure for more mechanization. The use of computers will become more widespread, facilitating the control of infection as well as the handling of results in the laboratories.

New techniques will be introduced. I expect that new methods will be applied to the recognition of infections caused by anaerobic organisms. Much attention will be paid to the detection of bacterial or viral antigens in clinical material from which it has not been possible to grow organisms. This may also be used as a means of speeding diagnosis. There will continue to be much development in rapid diagnostic techniques generally.

One of the most striking changes in clinical microbiology in recent years has been the escape of medical microbiologists from their laboratories. They are now to be found everywhere in the hospitals: in wards, in clinics, in sterile supply units, in the kitchens, among the domestic staff, in the pharmacy, and in the special units. They interpret their rôle as involvement in the prevention of infection, in the control of established infection, and in the diagnosis and treatment of infected patients. In the U.K., medical microbiologists are diversifying out of their laboratories into clinical practice, while in the U.S.A. communicable diseases physicians are moving in the opposite direction. A number of microbiologists in the U.K. now run clinics for patients with infections, and the question of microbiologists having charge of the care of hospital inpatients is increasingly under debate.

As I have suggested in earlier chapters, there is much work to be done in infection control in our hospitals with new problems constantly arising. These problems occur partly because of the introduction of new clinical procedures such as transplant surgery, neonatal intensive care, reconstructive vascular surgery or the use of central venous catheters: a process of innovation which may be expected to continue. Problems also arise because of the recognition of 'new', potentially transmissible infections such as Legionnaire's disease. There clearly will be a need for increased provision of isolation facilities in hospitals, and these will also be required to help in containing the spread of bacteria carrying unwelcome antibiotic resistances. There is also much scope, in my opinion, for clinical microbiologists to interest themselves in what goes on in general practice.

Changes in the field of antibiotics can be confidently expected in the years to come, because change has been ceaseless since the introduction of the first antimicrobial agents more than fifty years ago. I do not expect to see groups of fundamentally new drugs introduced, except perhaps in the field of antiviral chemotherapy; rather, there will be new variants of existing antibiotics with marginal advantages over existing products. The number of these will continue to increase, and increasing demands will be made on those with a special interest in antimicrobial chemotherapy to assist in the rational choice of treatment. Problems caused by antibiotic resistance in pathogenic organisms will continue to increase. In the previous chapter I discussed what might happen, if the bacteria or if man wins the battle of antibiotic resistance. I indicated that, in my opinion, man could win provided that he had the will to organize himself. While I am optimistic about this in the long term, I suspect that the situation will have to deteriorate much further before the political initiative is found to take the necessary action. In the short term, therefore, I am pessimistic enough to think that the successful use of antibiotics is going to become much more difficult. I hope that my anxieties about this may prove to be misplaced since the price in lost health or lives that will otherwise have to be paid is high.

A new development, just beginning, is 'genetic engineering'. This technique of implanting the genetic determinants of a characteristic in the nucleic acid of a host species so that it develops a desired new property is exciting in its potential. A recent development has been the transfer to *Escherichia coli* of the genetic material which codes for the production of human insulin. The bacteria now produce insulin more suitable than the animal insulins for use by diabetics. It may be that interferon will be produced by similar techniques in years to come, with unforeseeable results in promoting research in the prevention or treatment of viral infections and cancers. It is not possible to predict how such techniques will be developed, but the rate of change will be rapid and the developments may be even more unlikely sounding than the products of the imagination of past science fiction writers.

The nature of existing and expected challenges indicates to me that there can be no more exciting field of medical practice than clinical microbiology. Yet there are great difficulties in the UK in recruiting young doctors into the speciality. I suspect that this is because the subject is badly taught to medical students as a dry-as-dust discipline of little clinical relevance. In fact, it could scarcely be more relevant to successful clinical practice in any field. It will be very important in the years to come to change the pattern of undergraduate teaching. Students may then come to realize that clinical microbiology not only has a fascinating past but is full of wide ranging medical interest at present and promises exciting challenges for the future.

References

Andrewes, C. and Pereira, H. G. (1972). *Viruses of Vertebrates*. (London: Baillière Tindall)

Cowan, S. T. and Steel, K. J. (1974). *Cowan and Steel's Manual for the Identification of Medical Bacteria*. (London and New York: Cambridge University Press)

Grüneberg, R. N. (1979). The microbiological rationale for the combination of sulphonamides with trimethoprim. *J. Antimicrob. Chemother.*, **5** (Suppl. B), 27

Grüneberg, R. N. and Bendall, M. J. (1979). Hospital outbreak of trimethoprim resistance in pathogenic coliform bacteria. *Br. Med. J.*, **2**, 7

Grüneberg, R. N. and Bettelheim, K. A. (1969). Geographical variation in serological types of urinary *Escherichia coli*. *J. Med. Microbiol.*, **2**, 219

Grüneberg, R. N., Emmerson, A. M., Prankerd, T. A. J. and Souhami, R. L. (1970). Antibacterial prophylaxis in leukaemic neutropaenia using trimethoprim-sulphamethoxazole. *Proceedings of the Vth International Congress of Infectious Diseases*, Vienna, **3**, 387

Hill, M. J. *et al.* (1971). Bacteria and aetiology of cancer of large bowel. *Lancet*, **1**, 95

Howie, J. (1979). *Code of Practice for the Prevention of Infection in Clinical Laboratories and Post-mortem Rooms* [report of a working party]. (London: HMSO)

Howie, J. G. R. and Hutchison, K. R. (1978). Antibiotics and respiratory illness in general practice: prescribing policy and work load. *Br. Med. J.*, **2**, 1342

Leigh, D. A., Grüneberg, R. N. and Brumfitt, W. (1968). Long-term follow-up of bacteriuria in pregnancy. *Lancet*, **1**, 603

Modr, Z. (1978). Antibiotic policy in Czechoslovakia. *J. Antimicrob. Chemother.*, **4**, 305

173

Price, D. J. E. and Sleigh, J. D. (1970). Control of infection due to *Klebsiella aerogenes* in a neurosurgical unit by withdrawal of all antibiotics. *Lancet*, **2**, 1213

Richmond, M. H. and Linton, K. B. (1980). The use of tetracycline in the community and its possible relation to the excretion of tetracycline-resistant bacteria. *J. Antimicrob. Chemother.*, **6**, 33

Ridgeway, G. L. (1980). The chemotherapy of gonorrhoea and non-specific genital infections. In Grüneberg, R. N. (ed.) *Antibiotics and Chemotherapy: Current Topics*, Chap. 5. (Lancaster: MTP)

Shanson, D. C. (1980). The chemotherapy of infective endocarditis. In Grüneberg, R. N. (ed.) *Antibiotics and Chemotherapy: Current Topics.* Chap. 1. (Lancaster: MTP)

Smellie, J. M., Grüneberg, R. N. and Katz, G. (1978). Controlled trial of prophylactic treatment in childhood urinary-tract infection. *Lancet*, **2** 175

Stokes, E. J., Howard, E., Peters, J. L., Hackworthy, C. A., Milne, S. E. and Witherow, R. O. (1977). Comparison of antibiotic and antiseptic prophylaxis of wound infection in acute abdominal surgery. *World J. Surg.* **1**, 777

Swann, M. M. (1969). *Joint Committee on the Use of Antibiotics in Animal Husbandry and Veterinary Medicine* [Command Paper No. 4190]. (London: HMSO)

Symmers, W. St C. (1973). Amphotericin pharmacophobia. *Br. Med. J.*, **4**, 460

Threlfall, E. J. *et al.* (1980). Plasmid-encoded trimethroprim resistance in multiresistant epidemic *Salmonella typhimurium* phage types 204 and 193 in Britain. *Br. Med. J.*, **280**, 1210

Index

abortion
  and rubella 48
  spontaneous 16
advertising 129, 131
aerobes 23, 26
amphotericin B 54, 55, 61
ampicillin 15
  overuse and resistance 83
  use and urinary pathogen
    sensitivity 63, 64
anaerobes 23, 26
anamnestic response 30, 32
animal husbandry and antibiotic use
  65, 160—2
anthrax 121
antibiotics
  administration 76—8
  adverse reactions 59—61
  agricultural use 65, 160—2
  antibacterial 59—83
  antifungal 54, 55
  bactericidal and bacteristatic,
    roles 71, 72
  black market and controls 160,
    161
  combinations 72—4
  constraints on choice 59—67

control of 151—63
cost 65—7, 80, 81, 83, 141
dosing 77, 78
drug choice 78, 79
experts on 81
minimum inhibitory
    concentration 77
and mixed infections 73
monitoring 70, 71, 82
prescribing policies 159
prophylaxis 74—6, 83, 102
resistance 25, 61—5, 75, 79, 80
restrictions on use 76, 77, 157—9,
  162
sensitivity 30, 68, 69
antibodies
  antibacterial 24
  changes in infection 48
  rubella IgM, significance 48
antigens
  bacterial O, K and H 23, 28
  HBsAg 49, 146, 148
Ascaris lumbricoides 56
aspergilloma 54
aspergillosis, invasive 54
Aspergillus spp. 51—4
australia antigen 49

bacilli   22, 26
bacteria
   accidental infections   11
   antibiotic sensitivity of urinary
      63
   cell wall   22, 23
   classification   26—28
   conjugation   24, 25, 62
   factors affecting growth   22, 23,
      26, 29, 73, 74
   folate metabolism   73, 84
   genetics   25
   Gram-negative in hospitals   101
   R factors   62
   resistance see antibiotics
   staining   26
   strain identification   28, 29
   tests   27—32
   toxins   23
bacteriocines   28
bacteriology laboratory   28—39,
      104, 105
   culture work   28—30
   growth in workload   169, 170
   infectious diseases   35—9
   monitoring   70, 71
   PUO investigations   36—9
   risks   33, 35, 146, 147
   routine screening   106, 107
   serology   30—2
   specimen collection for   32—5
   use of   86, 105—7
bacteriophages   25, 28
biopsy   39
blood transfusion   148
Bordetella pertussis immunization
      124
botulism   118
bronchitis   90
bronchopneumonia   90
brucellosis   16, 17, 35, 39, 118
Buruli ulcer   18

Campylobacter spp. enteritis   18,
      167

C. jejuni temperature optimum
      22
cancer and viruses   168
Candida albicans   52
Candida spp.   51, 102
   treatment   73
   vaginitis   15, 95
catheter hygiene   113, 114, 140, 148
cephalosporins   66, 67, 81
cetrimide   24
Chlamydia spp.   22, 41, 42, 167
chloramphenicol   72, 126
   limited use   60, 61
   resistance spread   152
cholera   92, 116, 117, 125, 167
Clostridium difficile colitis   18
   C. perfringens   91, 96
cocci   22, 26
colonization   19, 20
Corynebacterium diphtheriae   17
   lysis and diphtheria toxin   25, 44
   therapy   86
co-trimoxazole   61, 74, 90, 126
   composition   73
   prophylactic in immune deficiency
      110
   and trimethoprim resistance   154,
      155
   in urinary tract infections   67, 68,
      93, 94, 113
Cryptococcus neoformans   51, 52

diarrhoea, control of   92, 147
diphtheria   17, 25, 44, 123, 124
disease, notifiable   120, 136, 137
DNA
   bacterial   22, 25
   viral and classification   41, 42
dysentery   92

Ebola fever   18, 135, 146, 166
endocarditis, infective   35, 39
   and bactericidal drugs   71

diagnosis 108
  laboratory role 70
  organisms causing 108
  treatment monitoring 70, 108, 109
endometritis 96
endotoxins 23
Entamoeba histolytica 56
enteric fever 126, 137
  diagnosis 31
  treatment 92
Enterobius vermicularis 56
epidemics 13, 115
Epidermophyton floccosum 51, 52
erythrocyte sedimentation rate 37
Escherichia coli
  insulin production by 172
  intestinal tract virulence 44
  number in faeces 14
  serotyping 28
  urinary tract infection 14, 15, 159
exotoxins 23, 25
  food poisoning 91
  shock 108

fimbriae 24
flagella 22
5-fluorocytosine 55
food poisoning causes 91
fungi 50—5

gastro-intestinal infections in general practice 91, 92
genetic changes, bacteria and man 15
genetic engineering, insulin production 172
genito-urinary infection 94—6
gentamicin 61
  monitoring 70
  neonatal 111
gonorrhoea 16, 33
Gram-stain 26, 27

haemodialysis 148, 149
haemoglobin 37
Haemophilus spp. growth factors 23
  H. influenzae epiglottis 91
health education 129—31
helminths 55—8
hospital
  acquired infections, costs 134
  admission policy 134, 135
  burns unit, infections 149
  design of 135, 136
  infection control 133—50
  kitchens and infection 143, 145
  laboratory safety 146, 147
  occupational health of staff 144, 145
  operating theatre and infection 143
  paediatric management 147, 148
  patients, infections among 99—103, 152—8
  pest control 144
  pharmacy design 140, 141
  precautions 138, 139, 140
  prescribing policy 163
  sharp object disposal 145, 146
  sterile supply 141—3
  surveillance in 163
  ward closure 138
housing 130

immune deficiency 109, 110
immunization 122—28, 166, 167
  BCG 145
  cholera 125
  diphtheria 123
  enteric fever 166
  hospital staff 145
  influenza 127
  measles 127
  passive hepatitis 126, 146
  rabies 166
  research increase 166
  risks 124—28, 167

immunization (*continued*)
  rubella   48, 126, 145
  smallpox eradication and   123, 125
  TAB   32, 126
immunofluorescence   44
infections
  changing nature   13, 18, 167
  as clinical diagnosis   19
  and colonization   19, 20
  contact tracing   121, 122
  contaminant   120—22
  control in community   115—31
  control in hospitals   133—50
  in general practice   85—97
  in hospitals   99—114
  mixed, treatment   73
  non-specific, clinical features   17
  specific and primitive cultures   17
  surveillance   119, 120
inflammation   19
influenza   127
  antigenic types, emergence of 120, 128
  variation in   13, 127, 128
intensive care   147, 148
interferon   43
intravenous infusion   140
isolation   121, 137, 138

Koch's postulates   17, 18

Lassa fever   14, 18, 121, 135, 137, 146, 166
Legionella pneumophila   18, 167
leprosy   17, 18

Madurella mycetomi   53
malaria   13, 57
Marburg disease   18, 135, 166
measles   13, 127, 147
microbes   12—15
microbiology   11, 12, 165—72

Microsporum spp.   51, 52
multiple sclerosis   168
Mycobacterium leprae   17
  in armadillo   18
  M. ulcerans   18, 22
Mycobacterium tuberculosis
  generation time   24
Mycoplasma pneumoniae   89

Neisseria gonorrhoeae   16
  N. meningitidis carrier state   20

penicillin   75
  resistance   62, 152
  V, dose and haemolytic streptococci   88, 89
plague   13, 115, 116
plasmids   25
Plasmodium spp., identification   57
pneumonia, treatment of lobar   90
pollution and wandering tribes   11, 12
population growth projections   165, 166
povidone iodine   76
pregnancy
  antibiotics in   94
  and rubella   48, 49
prophylactic chemotherapy   74—5, 83, 102
protozoa   55—8
Pseudomonas aeruginosa   23, 24, 147
public health laboratories   91
pyrexia of unknown origin (PUO) 36—9

rabies   121
respiratory tract infections   88—91
ringworm   51
RNA   22, 41, 42

Salmonella spp.   167
  fermentation   29

serotypes 27
S. paratyphi 17
S. typhi 16, 17, 18, 20, 31, 118
S. typhimurium in animals 161
scarlet fever 13
Schistosoma spp. 56
screening, value of routine 106
septicaemia 107—111 *see also*
endocarditis
serology 28, 30—2, 47, 53, 58, 88
sewage treatment and disposal
117, 118
Shigella spp. 29, 92
sinusitis diagnosis 89
specimen collection 32—5, 71, 86,
87
spirochaetes 22, 26
staphylococcal enterocolitis 15
Staphylococcus aureus
bacteriophage typing 28
exotoxin 91
Streptococcus spp., group A
haemolytic 86, 96
and penicillin 61, 75, 88, 89
virulence 13
sulphonamide resistance 152
synergy 73, 74
syphilis 13, 32, 106

tapeworms 56
temperature and bacterial growth
22
tetracycline, adverse microbial
reaction 15
transduction 25, 62
transformation 25, 62
Trichomonas vaginalis 95
trimethoprim 152—8
tuberculosis eradication 166
typhoid fever 14, 16, 117, 119, 122,
161

urban development and disease 12
urinary tract infections
antibiotic ranking 67, 68
catheter-associated 113
features in hospital 100, 112—14
in general practice 93, 94
organisms causing 112
overdiagnosis 69
pathogen sensitivity 62—4
recurrent 93
treatment 65, 66, 113

vaginitis 15, 95
venereal disease 94, 95, 122
Vibrio cholerae 17
vibrios 22, 26
virulence 13
virus 18, 41—6, 48, 121
classification 42
culture 36, 87
and disease in man 168
electron microscopy 44, 45
in general practice 88
hepatitis 49, 145, 148
infection process 43
nucleic acid types 41, 42
quiescent 43, 44
respiratory syncytial 44, 90
serology 47, 48
size and symmetry 41, 42
smallpox 16, 18, 46, 123, 137, 146
tissue culture 42, 46, 47

water, clean 116—18
whooping cough 24
Widal test 31, 32
wound dressing 101
infections 111, 112
treatment 97, 111, 112, 139

yeasts 50

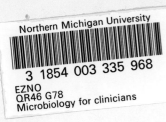